UNDERSTANDING LIFE BACKWARDS

2

UNDERSTANDING LIFE BACKWARDS

A memoir

Tim Cartmill AO

Lorikeet Press, 2023

UNDERSTANDING LIFE BACKWARDS

First edition. May 9, 2023

ISBN: 978-0-6454625-2-4
Written by Tim Cartmill AO FRACS

Foreword

What a privilege to be asked to provide this foreword to my father's memoir! Somewhat taciturn and usually at work like many of his contemporaries at that time, this pioneering children's heart surgeon was a stranger to me for much of my childhood, though always ready to engage in philosophical discussions with great insight, good humour and breadth of perspective if specifically asked.

This memoir fills in many gaps in my knowledge and confirms that Tim's life-saving work kept him more than busy night and day. Stern silences I may once have interpreted as disapproval or disinterest were more likely to have been due to exhaustion and frustrations about political decisions at the highest levels as he did his best to influence change for the better.

Either way, Tim's succinct style, razor sharp analysis and dry wit make for a riveting read, while he sheds light on Australian life, medical breakthroughs and global events. Tim has made the most of his opportunities to improve the lives of so many others.

Born in tight times during the wake of the Great Depression, Timothy Boyd Cartmill spent his early life as a curious, barefoot farm boy who loved to read and learn. He caught the attention of the teacher at his tiny school, and earned a State Bursary to Hurlstone Agricultural High School, a selective State boarding school. After breaking a collarbone wrestling with his brother and discovering the value of the work of doctors, Tim went on to study Medicine at the University of Sydney. He met and later married my mother, nursing student then theatre nurse and dedicated wife, mother and homemaker, Marilyn McKenzie, in the 1950s.

Tim operated and studied in Sydney and the US, supporting his young family, then returned to Australia, where he worked all hours at multiple hospitals, while taking on honorary representative roles with his hospital and surgical associations.

Later chapters address his work in developing countries and the Arabian Gulf, tackled with the same curiosity, energy and taste for travel which characterised his early life.

Tim's reflections and warm acknowledgement of mentors and colleagues hint at a humility and abiding sense of wonder at the world.

In the appendices, the clarity of Tim's descriptions of experimental heart surgery and treatments contribute fascinating historical records, while his reflections on technological innovation and politics are elucidating.

I embrace this opportunity to thank and congratulate him on his extraordinary achievements, including his creation of *Understanding Life Backwards*, this useful and entertaining resource for a wide audience.

Alison Handmer (nee Cartmill)

Contents

8

Introduction

Life can only be understood backwards; but it must be lived forwards.
Søren Aabye Kierkegaard: *Journals IV* A 164 (1843)

As I grow older, I feel more the need to integrate the experiences of my life, to find patterns of connection in them that tie me to family, to community. – Gino Segre Einstein's *Refrigerator* page 272

I am writing this memoir mainly for my family and a few friends. I hope to reflect on selected important experiences, with emphasis on those I enjoyed and what I think I learned from them.

I sometimes use the term "waypoints" to describe important life events that led to changes in direction, significant advances in knowledge or experience, and unexpected developments. It is not a perfect analogy. A navigator generally selects waypoints in advance whereas a memoirist recognises them in hindsight, often long after the fact.

Many of my waypoints involve other people, especially teachers: they must have due prominence.

Chapter 1: Youth and education

The first 16 years

I am a farm boy, sprung from a long line of farmers. I was born in South Grafton on the Clarence River in northern New South Wales on 10 May 1933, second child and first son of Archie Everard John Cartmill and Emma Wilhelmine Cartmill nee Unwin.

Cartmills and McCaughys (my paternal grandmother's family name) were Northern Irish Protestants, among the millions who emigrated to Australia and elsewhere at the time of the potato blight in mid 19C. Thomas and Rosann Cartmill arrived in Sydney in 1853 and Thomas was employed as a shepherd near Armidale, NSW. They later tried their luck at the gold diggings near Uralla, before moving in 1863 with their growing family to settle at Skinner's Swamp on the then route from Grafton, NSW, to the tablelands. Thomas and his sons became bullock teamsters, settling on small farms on which they made their homes, grew some crops and raised their cattle. My Grandfather, John Cartmill, later moved down the creek from Skinner's Swamp, first nearer the present Armidale Road, thence to the "Eight-Mile", where the current Grafton-Armidale Road crosses Blaxland's Creek (so called because it was that distance from the original "Nymboida" Station). Here John Cartmill raised his growing family, expanded his holdings and ran a general store.

Around 1906 the family moved the short distance inland to Nymboida and took over an existing hotel business including the original farm house, additional family accommodation, hotel rooms, bars, parlours and some storage. Separate buildings held a butcher shop, a general store, a public dance hall, a fine slab barn of the original farm which still stands, plus stables and sheds, a smithy and assorted outbuildings, stockyards, sties and dairy.

All these endeavours supported the numerous enterprises with which my grandfather John Cartmill occupied his large and still unmarried family. A 100- acre cultivation on the river flat was planted with maize. A growing herd of ruby-red Devon cattle grazed on surrounding freehold and leased acreage. Bullock teams were used to haul pine logs to the wharves in South Grafton, to cart goods as back-loading for the store and the hotel, and for contracting work such as road building. John even had an agency for an undertaking business, and hence did some coffin making. Evidently a lively and ambitious spirit, he eventually overreached himself and was caught out being owed several bad debts in the Great Depression. He died after a stroke, before I was born.

My maternal grandmother, Margaret McAulay, was part of the Free Scots Presbyterian Church community on the lower Clarence River. Her husband William John Unwin was an English migrant farm worker who married the boss's daughter.

My mother, Emma Unwin, was intelligent and strong-willed, born and raised on a sugarcane and dairy farm on Goodwood Island within the mouth of the Clarence River estuary. The primary school teacher used collect the nearby children from the island and row them across the channel to Wombah on the mainland for each school day.

Emma's secondary schooling was in the City of Grafton, requiring a weekly boat trip and boarding during each week. She attended Sydney Teachers College for the one-year course, traveling by coastal steamer as the railway had not yet reached Grafton. Few farm children had much schooling beyond Primary level at that time; certainly none of her siblings.

After graduation her first posting was to Blaxland's Creek, which she said she assumed was in the Blue Mountains. In fact, it was on the Armidale Road, near the area we called the Eight-Mile.

On the way to take up her posting she was held up at the flooded Orara River and had to be ferried across by boat. On the far side of the torrent, she was met by my father in his role of service car driver. [Motor transport was still developing at that stage, and Mail Cars, Service Cars, and sometimes dual- purpose cream lorries provided regular transport beyond the railheads and major towns.]

After lengthy familial skirmishing reflecting the clash of values between the strictly teetotal Scottish Unwins and the pub-owning Irish Cartmills, Archie and Emma were married in 1928. My sister Poppy was born in 1929 and I followed in 1933, thence my brother Gaine in 1936 and Rosemary in 1940.

We occupied a small cottage adjacent to the Hotel, separate from the living quarters of the rest of the family. I barely remember our grandma, Mary Ann (nee McCaughy), a domineering black-clad widowed matriarch who by then ruled mostly from her room. Our uncles and aunts, all remaining single, probably because their mother found all suitors unsuitable, formed an eccentric but affectionate and protective extended family.

As children we were on good terms with one another, though not very close as our ages were widely spaced. Our universe was the farm, the pub, and our own close family. We ate separately from the aunts and uncles except for about once a week and for feast days like Christmas.

By the time I remember, the main agricultural activities included corn (maize) production on the river flat, and beef cattle raising both around the farm and on bush country in neighbouring valleys, much of it leased.

Timber became an important cash crop during the Second World War, when squared timber was in demand for projects such as Garden Island dockyard in Sydney.

Dad and his brothers parcelled out responsibilities for these activities. Jim was the cattle expert, Owen contributed to cattle work and farming and was a skilful blacksmith and carpenter, Reg looked after general maintenance and roustabout duties, but teamed up with Dad for corn planting. In fact, all of them pitched in for the work at hand. Dad, as youngest son and having completed schooling to age fourteen, was the only fully literate one of the boys, and the brains of the outfit. He was licensee of the pub after his mother's death and spent a fair proportion of his time on the business. He also was the driver, and in the early years ran a car service to Grafton each Tuesday, taking that opportunity to conduct business in town.

The maiden aunts had their tasks; Daisy, the eldest, worked every day in the kitchen at the great wood cooking range, while Gladys was in charge of the bar. In early days that was often only busy at peak times, such as cattle sales which were held in our yards. As industries such as a sawmill and a local coalmine waxed and waned, there were busy times as the men knocked off from work. Saturday was a time for the locals to gather, play cards, and listen to the horse races on the big six-valve superheterodyne wireless set, turned up loud.

Our family members always took their civic responsibilities seriously. My father and mother were leaders in school, community, church matters, committees, associations and charities and regularly served as office bearers. These activities are the glue that keeps small communities together. They gave satisfaction to the participants, helped the needy, and contributed to necessary developments. As they say, "History is made by those who turn up".

"T'was Mulga Bill from Eaglehawk that caught the cycling craze
And turned away the good old horse that served him many days..."

Banjo Paterson's "Mulga Bill's Bicycle" was our very favourite poem for Mum to read by the open fire on cold winter nights after supper. The cottage had almost no insulation and the nights grew frosty fast, so the hot open fire was at a premium. The bed of hardwood coals hissed and sputtered and the flames burst out, as we clustered round for the evening reading. During winter Mother always cooked over that open fire on a couple of iron bars fashioned from an old cart tyre flattened out in the forge for the purpose. Good enough to hold a frying pan, a pot or two and a black kettle. With luck the embers smouldered until morning.

Not only the absurd antics of Mulga Bill, but the Canon of Australian Bush Poets, as well as short stories — all these were our intellectual substrate. The Brothers Grimm, and Longfellow (those were names for a child to ponder); also a good sampling of Palgrave, and I suppose Walter Scott, Henry Lawson and the unrelated Will Lawson, the Banjo, Tennyson, Jack London. *Hiawatha, A Bush Christening, Said Hanrahan, The Loaded Dog, Huck Finn and Tom Sawyer, Harry Dale, The Little Red Hen, The Three Little Pigs* ... What emotional fodder for youngsters, and what better way to learn to love books and writing, even before we had learned to read.

Replete with dinner, drowsy with the reading and the hypnotic fire, our coarse flannel pyjamas toasted by the coals, it was time for a quick dash to the verandah and into our icy sheets. A few convulsive shivers, a snuggle, and off to sleep, still tickled by Mulga Bill's spectacular downfalls.

"*...a horse's back is good enough henceforth for Mulga Bill.*"

While Mum was unfailing at reading aloud, Dad favoured reciting from memory his school stories. Charles Lamb's "*Roast Pig*" was a favourite, beginning: "*Ho-Tai and his son, Bo-Bo, a great lubberly lad ...*"

There was always something to read in our house. Dad and Mum habitually read periodicals such as *The Australian Women's Weekly* and *Smith's Weekly*, as well as the Grafton *Daily Examiner* newspaper. Even comic books were bought when we were old enough to appreciate them. They may be lowbrow but comics are another good way for children to enter the world of words. *The Phantom*, *Ginger Meggs*, and *Buck Rogers* were personal favourites. We also had a good-sized bookshelf containing the books which my mother had collected as a student.

Within the hotel there was a small dark room, known as the private parlour, used only for such events as drinks before the Christmas dinner. On the wall was a glass-fronted cedar book case containing a few dozen volumes. I probably found David Copperfield there and Charles Kingsley's *The Water Babies*.

About that time, just when I was ready for it, my aunt Gladys purchased Arthur Mee's *The Children's Encyclopaedia*. I suppose it was pressed on her by a travelling salesman, because her own reading rarely extended beyond the local newspaper. The Encyclopaedia consisted of ten or a dozen handsome red volumes, smartly produced and printed with plenty of illustrations on good paper, and held in their own little pine bookshelf. Just the thing for an avaricious reader hungry for material!

This Encyclopaedia was not set out in the usual form of alphabetically listed essays under various learned headings, but each volume was subdivided into many sections covering topics as diverse as: Myths and Legends, Ancient History, Children and People of Many Lands, How Things Work, Things to Make and Do and many other topics. It was ideal for browsing, and had a good index, making it a useful reference source.

Many a happy hour I spent in that gloomy room under a dim electric bulb to illuminate one of those books spread out on the heavily covered table, and with my mind far away. Heavy books for a bookish boy! Aunty Gladys probably read hardly a single page of them. Once in a while she would drop in to enjoy the sight of my enjoyment. I remain very much in her debt for allowing me the chance to read such solid material so soon.

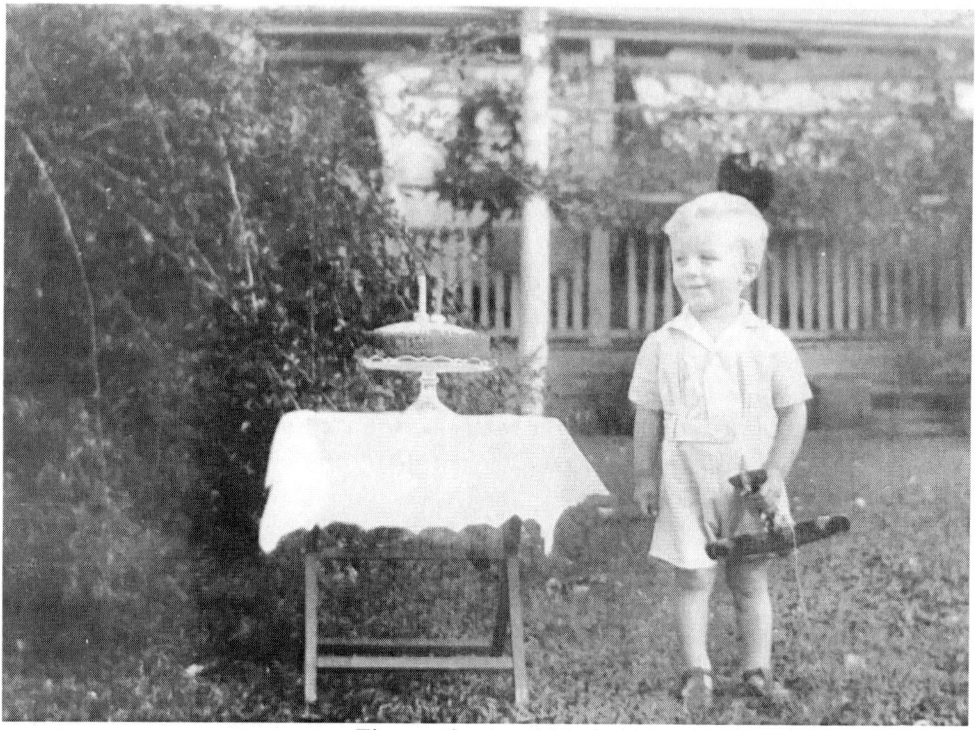

Tim aged two at Nymboida

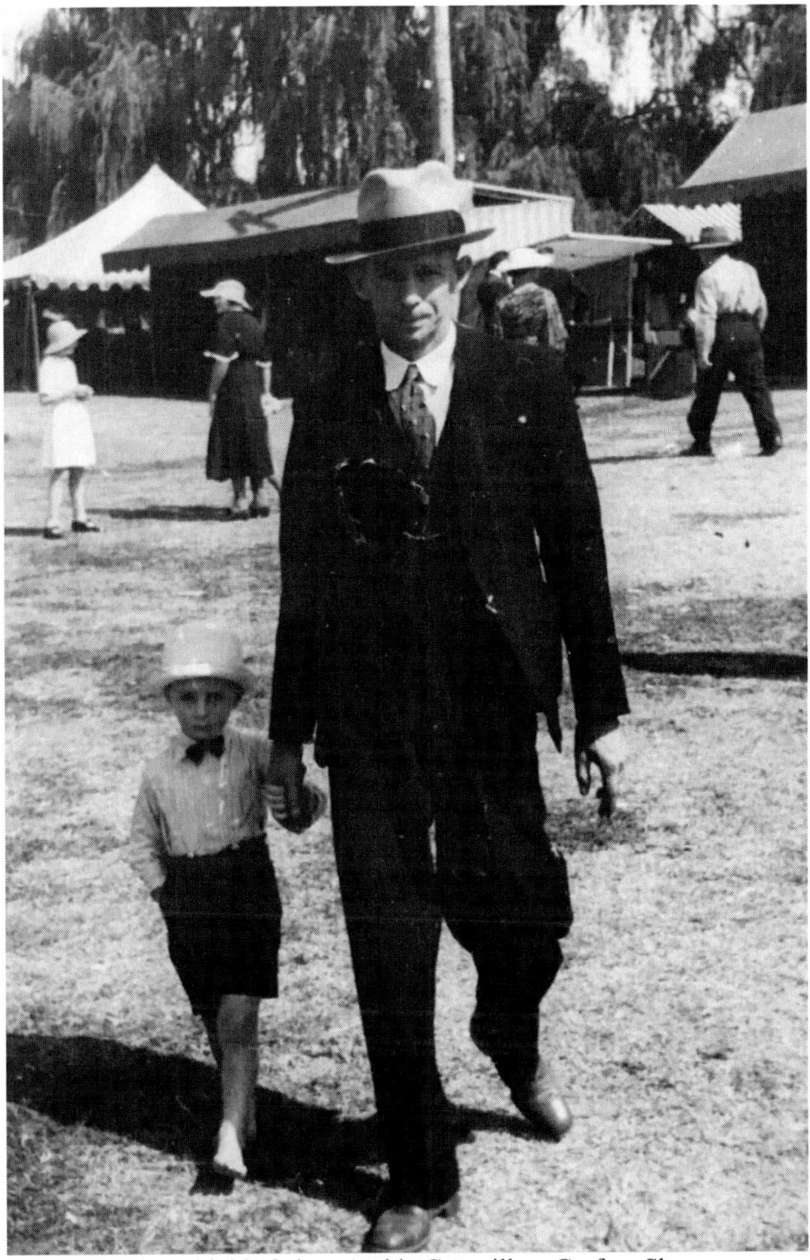
Tim with his father, Archie Cartmill, at Grafton Show

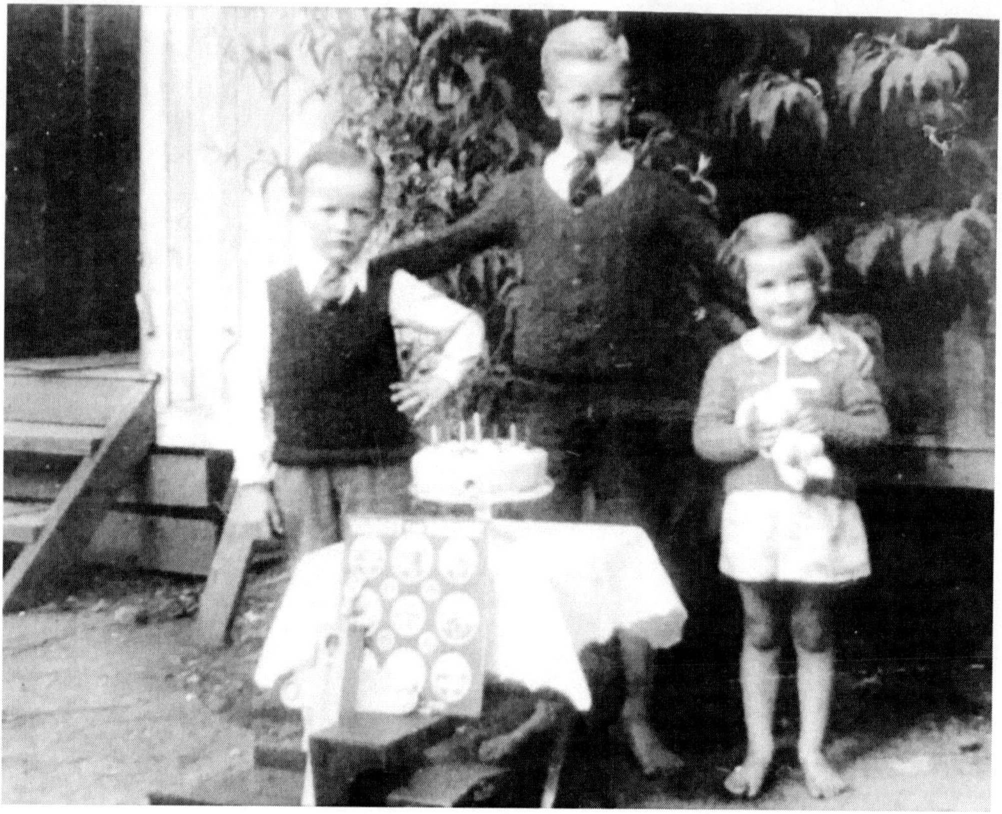

Tim with younger siblings, Gaine (left) and Rosemary

Nymboida Primary School

I started school at age five years and eight months, I suppose because I was "bright" and my mother was keen and ambitious for me and my sibs, and had the professional engagement of a former teacher. I set off with my new shirt and shorts and straw hat (no shoes), and was invited by the teacher Mr Chambers to nominate an older boy to be my friendly supporter. I chose a good looking chap a couple of years my senior, called Basil. I had met him before, he seemed okay, and he wore a round topped felt hat.

Basil was helpful at first, but he later joined the others in bullying me. I cannot remember why, but I was such a small, skinny young kid that I would have been a suitable target. Basil's main claim to fame later was that he was the only boy to wear shoes in winter. This gave him a decided advantage in soccer, and he always kept his shoes on so he never had to wash his feet, he said.

Nymboida had a typical country one-room school house (actually there were two rooms but only one was in use in my time, as there were only between about 20 and 30 pupils. Later, when the local coal mine was working at its peak, there were a few more children and local girl, Patty Clark, returned from college to teach for some years). Classes were Years 1 to 6, with a couple of older girls making up a Year 7.

It was there I had the first of my many strokes of luck with teachers. At the first May vacation Mr Chambers was replaced by Mr Wal Baker, a recently graduated "young comer". A coalfields boy from Kurri Kurri, he was smart, ambitious, and athletic. His supposed Communist sympathies did not endear him to everyone and his fondness for the "German Music" of Beethoven even less so. He was simply a superb teacher, organised to keep all the levels functioning all the time. He developed such a reputation as a disciplinarian that renegades were sometimes shipped in from as far distant as Coutts' Crossing for taming.

A small collection of books in the vacant rear classroom served as library and held a few more advanced books, many of which I read. That is where I encountered Jules Verne's *Journey to the Moon*. Later I read *Journey Around the Moon* and then tried *20,000 Leagues Under the Sea*, but found it about 10,000 Leagues too long for me.

There was a good Education Department scheme whereby a wooden box arrived monthly by rail from a central library service in Sydney. The books were devoured by most of us and the box was exchanged each month for a fresh selection. A similar scheme distributed vinyl records, which were played on an old wind-up portable Gramophone machine which required a second cranking to maintain some speed toward the end of a 12-inch record. Scratchy no doubt, but an introduction to opera, operetta, hearty songs of Empire, and the dreaded Beethoven among many. I recall Caruso, *The Barber of Seville*, *The Marriage of Figaro*, *White Horse Inn* and Peter Dawson. Actually, I suspect the Beethoven might have been Mr Baker's own records and he played them at his residence in the school grounds, prudently using his own better-quality player. Primitive technology, but those old records, supplemented by *The Argonauts* on the ABC radio, were a great start to a lifelong love of amateur music appreciation.

Several children rode horses to school, left them in the horse paddock all day, and were let out of class a few minutes early to saddle up for the ride home. I cadged a lift to school three mornings a week with Budge McLennan in his lorry taking cream to the Grafton Norco butter factory, and with Dad on his regular run on Tuesdays, leaving only Thursday to walk the mile and a quarter. Afternoons we walked home in a straggling mob, often dawdling to skip stones or get up to mischief. As I got bigger, I preferred a loping jog, so I probably became pretty fit.

School sports were often variants of "chasings", such as Bobbies and Bushies, Tip You Last, or Cops and Robbers. Sometimes we played cricket with an old tennis ball but the clay pitch was terrible, so the softball-like game of Rounders using a broom handle and old tennis ball was preferred for summer. The Parents & Citizens Association donated a soccer ball and that provided a more organised game for winter. The disparity in size, gender and aptitude of the pupils was always a problem. In any case I had no talent for sport and therefore little interest, though I always tried.

By about Second or Third Class I had pushed ahead of the mob in Reading and had no trouble with Sums, so I got promoted to the next higher grade. Thus, by the time I repeated 6th year to be old enough for high school I had made a start on Algebra and was reading very well. At the end of Primary School in 1944, aged 11 years, I won a State Bursary and was able to graduate to the selective State boarding school, Hurlstone Agricultural High School at Glenfield, near Liverpool in Sydney.

Footnote on Mr Wal Baker

This ambitious and excellent teacher advanced rapidly through the ranks, eventually becoming Headmaster at Maitland.

I next encountered him in the early 1990s when I was consulted about him while he was a patient in Ryde Hospital suffering bacterial endocarditis, a potentially lethal infection of a heart valve, apparently resistant to all antibiotic therapy.

I had Wal transferred to Westmead Hospital, where I carried the unpalatable responsibility of performing a very high-risk operation to remove the mitral valve and replace it with an artificial prosthesis, in the face of uncontrollable infection.

In the nick of time our Infectious Diseases gurus managed to find an effective drug and I was off the hook. Mr Baker and I enjoyed many chats as he recovered. Sadly, a few years later he developed motor neurone disease.

High school

It was inevitable that I would go to High School. My mother's conviction, with which I certainly agree, was that education is the main route to self-improvement, and the way in which those with reasonable intelligence could escape from a rural environment. I had shown aptitude in primary school by jumping a class and thus being so young that I had to repeat the final year anyway. But, why Hurlstone Agricultural High?

My elder sister, Poppy, had won a bursary and gone to Armidale High School, and, come to think of it, I do not know why the family chose there rather than Grafton. Probably it had a better academic record or maybe a better reputation. There was some difficulty with Poppy's accommodation though, and she became very unhappy with the church hostel at which she was staying, but later boarded with the family of a school friend.

Perhaps more decisive in my case was the fact that Bill Brown, one year my senior, whose father was a maintenance man at the local power station, had gone to Hurlstone with a scholarship. Hurlstone had two outstanding qualities: it was a selective high school, and also one of the few State boarding schools, the others being Farrer Agricultural High School at Tamworth, and Yanco at Temora in the Riverina. My State Bursary made Hurlstone financially possible as it covered boarding, tuition and some expenses for books and travel.

Getting kitted out was part of the big adventure. So many shirts, so many pairs of trousers, so many socks, etc. The heavy leather work boots were a new experience; indeed, at primary school we rarely wore shoes at all, except on the frostiest mornings. Each item had to be identified with a carefully sewn Cash's name tape (not the boots!). [These nametags were ordered from Sydney and arrived as a roll of cotton tape mechanically embroidered with the name in bright red or blue lettering. Mine were RED CAPS. Mother neatly sewed the labels into a neckband or waistband and they were an effective and tidy alternative to "indelible" ink, which always ran.]

Mum and I travelled to Sydney on the North Coast mail train, an exciting new experience for me as I had never been on a train. After the 15-hour trip to

Sydney we arrived next morning weary and dirty, but were taken in by Mum's old Sydney Teachers' College friend Rita Reid, who lived in Haberfield. Next morning, we caught the suburban electric to Liverpool, where we changed to the little steam train to semi-rural Glenfield.

School was a real eye opener for a Bushy like me. Everything was on a grand scale, the buildings, the crowds, even the senior boys who towered above us Freshers. We spent a long day waiting on the verandah of the admin building for admission proceedings to be completed. It was there that I met Bruce Cockerell and his mother. Bruce and I remained close friends through school.

Somewhere in that long day, Mum disappeared and the school routine began. Wake up in our twelve-bed dorm to a bell (the school's siren was reserved for air raids even at that late time in the War), sketchy ablutions, rushed breakfast of cereal, fresh milk and brown sugar and tea in the dining room, return to make beds for inspection, and so to class.

In the first couple of years each class had its separate "portable" classroom, a decrepit demountable building down the hill from the main brick structures. Classes got under way and we met our new teachers.

Classes began at about half past eight, giving time for the "Dagoes" (Day Boys) to arrive by the quarter past eight train. (By contrast, the boarders were, equally disparagingly, called "Bedbugs"). Each period was of 40 minutes. At mid-morning we had recess, when the lucky few who were cashed-up might buy some food at the tuck shop, followed by a couple more periods until lunch.

Lunch of roast meat, often mutton, with spuds and maybe some other vegetable and a simple dessert, was taken in the dining room by the boarders, and was the main meal of the day. More classes for the afternoon, then an exodus of the day boys, while the boarders rushed to queue up for the daily ration of "slabs and bog". The slab was a generous end-crust of wholemeal bread, while bog was the colloquial and scatological term applied to the thin scrape of raspberry jam applied thereto. We were hungry enough by four o'clock to eat the simple food with relish (more accurately, with bog).

There followed the ritual of mail call, when the senior student mounted the rear steps of the kitchen and called out the names of those lucky enough to receive a letter. Mum wrote every week, and I would reply, however cryptically. [I never had much to say.]

That left time for organised or informal sport until teatime, when we had a simple meal, usually of leftovers and some bread and jam. There was more time for outside activity before the start of Prep at seven o'clock, lasting for two hours with a short break at half time. Lights-out was at ten o'clock. That was the routine week in week out except in final year when the students preparing for their Leaving Certificate continued a later Prep in the library adjacent to the dining room, broken by a nice late supper of toast, jam and tea.

Our school participated in the Combined High Schools competitions in cricket, rugby football, and I think swimming. In general, we performed well, particularly in rugby. The organised sports day was Wednesday afternoon, when we travelled to other schools, or in the case of swimming, to Granville pool, always by train. Less formal sports included soccer, softball, and, always, French cricket or, even better, "gets out goes in" cricket, in which there are no teams, but whoever gets a dismissal becomes the next batsman, while the less talented spend a lot of time fielding. Thus we spent endless hours in the evenings and at weekends.

On Saturday afternoon we were allowed to go to the pictures, either at Ingleburn or in Liverpool. The movies were very popular entertainment at that time because there was so little else. The show included some blurred and dusty advertising slides, a newsreel or two showing mostly heavily censored war stories, a couple of cartoons like *Donald Duck* or *Road Runner*, a B-class movie and then, after the interval, the feature film. I suppose we saw most of the Hollywood films of the day. Audience participation included a fair amount of hooliganism and rowdiness, and a good time was had by all. If we had some money we would often buy a steak and eggs on the way back to the train, a valuable supplement to a pretty sketchy diet.

Everyone was required to go to church or Sunday school in the village. We Presbyterians, of whom there were not many, used walk to Glenfield Presbyterian Church for service in the afternoon. In time, most of us underwent a conversion of convenience to attend the Anglican service, because it was held at eleven o'clock, was well finished before lunch, and indeed was more easily wagged if one chose to go swimming in the George's River instead. The only memorable enlightenment which I gained from these organised religious activities came from one of the local worthies, Mr Kennett, who occasionally delivered a sermon in the Presbyterian church as a lay preacher. I still remember the text from Ecclesiastes 9:10: "*Whatsoever thy hand findeth to do, do it with thy might; for there is no work, nor device, nor knowledge, nor wisdom, in the grave, whither thou goest*". It has in fact been an important message for life.

High School teachers

Most of our teachers were excellent, no doubt because ours was a selective high school. This was the place for educational movers and shakers, several of whom were destined to become leading lights in the State's education system. Several older teachers who had stayed on because of the War had a weary Mister Chips quality about them. We had a share of green beginners and a few successful sportsmen, who were naturally attractive to the boys. Tall, blonde and handsome Keith Tull was still playing Rugby for the Sydney University Club, and coached our First Grade team for some years. A few of the unmarried teachers lived in their own semi-detached cottage adjacent to our dormitory block and supervised the boarders after school hours.

I must mention a few of the more memorable staff members:

The headmaster when I began was Mr Hindmarsh. He was very well liked and admired by the boys because he was a fair minded and open man, and had a huge enthusiasm for school sports, especially Rugby.

His deputy, Stanley Cook, was one of those bustling fat men in a tight suit, and was known, not affectionately, as the Runt, the unloved, unprepossessing and unpromising smallest member of a sow's litter. One reason that we didn't like Stanley very much what that he was responsible for discipline, and hence the most formal and frequent user of the cane. He did a good job as master in charge of the Dairy. He attended every morning, winter and summer from six o'clock and supervised the milking, feeding the cows, chilling the milk and even brewing the coffee. That coffee was made with pure, fresh Ayrshire milk, sweetened with brown sugar, and tasted mighty good with a large slab of toast slathered with dripping and sprinkled with coarse salt. I was never in one of the Runt's maths classes. He was a prominent Anglican, supporting the local church. More significantly, he had a couple of comely daughters, of whom the elder played the organ in church and for a while formed a choir singing hymns in the school. That accounted for one of the very few periods in my life when I showed sincere interest in religious matters.

After the first year, Hindmarsh was replaced by James McEwan King, a white-haired, patriarchal, upstanding and very decent Presbyterian. His wife, Millie, served as Matron and Cook in those frugal years immediately after the War, and Mr and Mrs King gave their all to keep the show running.

Harry Allen, known to all as Old Josh, was my Maths master through almost the whole of High School. He left for a short period somewhere in the middle but soon returned to take the top Maths classes. He was the quintessential chalky, who always wore the same old brown sports jacket and grey pants. Tall and skinny with a pointy nose, he would prowl into the room, sniff the air, declare that much more ventilation was needed (and considering the summer temperature of the old school rooms and the nature, social deportment and personal hygiene of the inhabitants, he was probably correct), then ostentatiously open all the windows before proceeding with the lesson.

He was a disciplinarian but never required force to maintain it. He could be tough on slackers. I still remember many of the lessons. While expounding on the pons asinorum, or Pythagoras' theorem, he would point out the benefits of cutting across the diagonal of a vacant corner block but said that "Stacey, who is a goat, would always walk the long way around". Stacey was a disruptive fidget in class. Allen had been a keen cricketer and coached First XI. One day, while the aforementioned Bob Stacey was mucking around and talking at the back of the class, Allen shied a duster at him. Stacey looked up just in time, caught the duster cleanly, and tossed it back to the teacher. "Good catch!" exclaimed Old Josh, "report to me at cricket practice immediately after school!"

Unfortunately, I was the only pupil interested in studying for Honours in Maths and it was decreed that we could not run a class for a single person. So my grasp of the integral calculus is still a bit sketchy.

Keith Pearson was a schoolboy's dream of a new-chum educator. An earnest Christian Fellowship type, tall, skinny and gawky, pictured best in his Scoutmaster's uniform as he exercised frail authority over his troop. The funny round hat, topping a narrow head with its jug ears and an oversized Adam's apple was set off by an incongruous neck scarf secured with a woggle made |of a sheep's vertebra. The uniform khaki shirt and generous Bombay bloomers showed off the skinny legs and knock knees to perfection, the ensemble underpinned by large flat shoes. Pearson was a decent chap, eager to please. One cold Easter I joined his Scouts camp as we headed off in the school's horse-drawn wagon to a campsite beside the George's River. Our Scout master taught us many useful things such as the bowline knot, and probably even more useless ones such as the sheepshank. I could sing some of the campfire songs even now if pressed. Unfortunately, in his role as camp cook Pearson managed to overshadow even the normal terrible standard of school food. Indeed, his stew condemned all of us to heavy-duty in the latrines.

Some of the prefects came to an informal agreement that this young teacher needed toughening up. Each evening when he supervised prep, they would send out a whole room, one row at a time, to receive the cane. Little damage was done to the pupils but, over time, the teacher's skill, force and accuracy improved. After a few months of this exercise, he became an accomplished wielder of the cane and was treated thereafter with a little more respect. Practice makes perfect!

Another mathematician by whom I was not regularly taught was Old Echo Wilcox. Maybe he got this odd nickname because his profound deafness resulted in a loud, flat-toned voice. More likely it was because he repeatedly announced, in the same voice, that he proposed to teach his classes "Economics, not to be confused with Bookkeeping which is a systematic and orderly method of keeping books". He wore a clumsy hearing aid, and a favourite torment was for his classes to speak gradually softer and softer to make him turn the amplifier louder and louder. Now with my own hearing challenges, I cringe to reflect that after the gain was at maximum it would be time to take a hexagonal pencil and roll it forcibly under the wooden desk to make a deafening noise in the earphones.

I enjoyed being taught French by Mr Westlake, imaginatively dubbed "Froggy" Westlake, a fine teacher, and like many of them an unapologetic enthusiast for all things French. Over five long years, we graduated from "la plume de ma tante" to "un bon vin blanc" and eventually to the subjunctive "si je perdais mon serin je serais très triste". No fault of Westlake's that I can still barely read a menu in French and just trust myself to ask the way to the bathroom.

Jim Peak was my most memorable English teacher. Under his guidance we even presented *A Midsummer Night's Dream* in a specially created outdoor amphitheatre carved on a sloping site using farm implements. The play, pretty ambitious for junior high school boys, was attended by many of the parents who lived not too far distant. Peak was one of the many teachers destined for great things in his profession.

Agriculture was a compulsory subject in our school and not too challenging. For most of the time our teacher was the very popular Bruce Gardner. After schooldays several of our class returned to the farm and many more contributed to the agricultural industry in one way or another; some went on to Hawkesbury Agricultural College, some studied Veterinary Science or Forestry, one continued his family's Friesian cattle breeding tradition and another eventually took over his family's farm machinery business in Nowra.

We also benefited indirectly from the lessons of some of the teachers in other classrooms. The fine blackboard diagrams left by the Botany teacher were so well remembered that I had little more to learn in that subject in first-year Medicine. Modern History was another topic, taken only by the non-mathematicians, that generated a lot of discussion and argument, which benefited all of us. Although the subject matter was mostly European History since the Middle Ages, much of Western culture came into play. If our timetable permitted, we would even sneak in to the back of that class.

At the end of 1949 I was looking forward to the Leaving Certificate examination. I had a good grasp of all the subjects with French being the only slightly wobbly one, and a sound technique for writing the papers. With just a few weeks to go, I and several of my friends developed chickenpox. We were quarantined in the small isolation cottage, no longer participated in class or prep, and were left to our own devices. The illness itself, although often thought of as a minor childhood illness, was quite debilitating.

Because of this, my final result in the Leaving Certificate exam was not as good as I had hoped as I only got second class Honours in English and a B in French and for the first time in all of school was not Dux of the class, being beaten at last by my good friend Richard Southern.

What I learned in high school

Boarding school can be a daunting experience for anybody, especially country children far from home. It is not for everyone; some could not tolerate the homesickness, loneliness and bullying. Some did not enjoy it much but held on somehow.

On balance, I found it a good experience and the source of many life skills. It planted a sense of self-sufficiency leading to self-reliance, physical and mental toughness, and ultimately stoicism and self-belief — all useful attributes for later life.

Hurlstone was my first exposure to a big institution in the larger world, with some serious academic competition. I consolidated my love of learning and appetite for competitive examinations. Above all I was exposed to many excellent teachers, learnt a great deal from all of them, and expected to proceed to higher education.

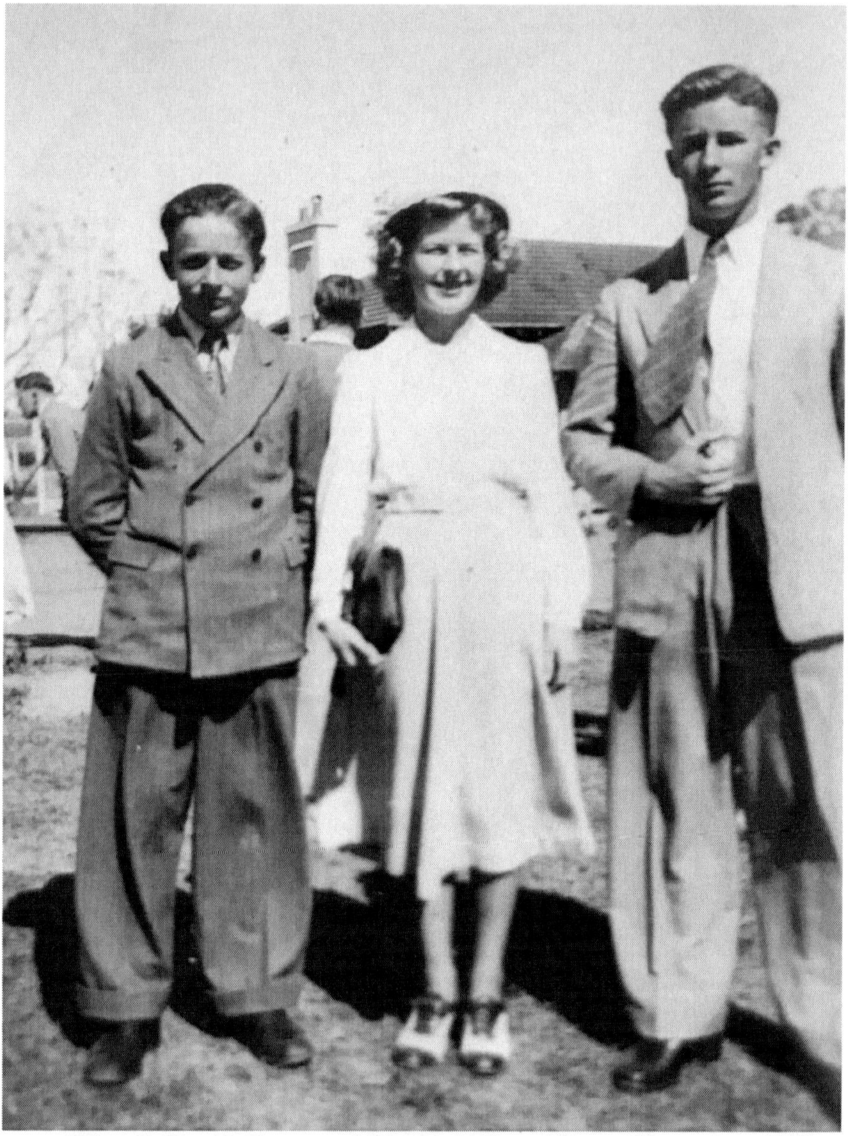

Gaine (left) with Poppy and Tim at the Royal Easter Show circa 1950

Chapter 2: Medical student years

"What will you be when you grow up?" Grown-ups often asked that question of children. I had no clear answer until my final year at High School. All academic work came easily to me and I was strongly attracted to science of some kind, without a clear understanding of what it entailed. For a while I favoured teaching, until it dawned on me that only a very few teachers get to teach the top class in Mathematics all the time. I didn't really want to return to the farm.

On my 16th birthday I had the good fortune to fracture my clavicle while wrestling with my brother. Gaine was younger but stronger and more athletic and we enjoyed such brotherly horseplay. This fracture was a minor one, but the hours that followed it were quite disabling. Painful, yes, and making every movement difficult. After what seemed quite a long time, the ambulance officers arrived from Grafton and applied the usual first-aid calico sling that was used in those days. The improvement was immediate and although there was still significant pain the feeling of instability was mostly gone. Having been transported to the Grafton Base Hospital I was cared for by the junior doctor on call, one Dr McGeoch. He replaced the triangular bandage sling with a more secure adhesive tape arrangement.

During follow-up visits young Dr McGeoch talked to me about career choices. He said he had begun to study Veterinary Science but switched to human Medicine instead. As I mused on the huge difference that medical and paramedical treatment could make in alleviating suffering, I came to think that this would be a worthwhile career.

St Andrew's College

Having graduated from High School with a reasonable Leaving Certificate pass, I was granted a State Bursary which allowed me to attend Sydney Medical School at the University of Sydney. On the recommendation of our local clergyman, the Rev Costello, it was decided that I would become a boarder at St Andrew's College within the University. Costello's son, Bill, was entering his final year of medical studies at college in that same year, 1950. [After training in Surgery at Royal Prince Alfred Hospital and further study in the UK, Bill Costello settled in Grafton for a long and successful career.]

St Andrew's had been established by the Presbyterian Church to accommodate country students. It was and is a fine institution, housed in a striking Scottish Gothic sandstone building within the University campus. The building was officially opened in 1876 and the first eight resident students moved in, including one who became a doctor.

Additional wings were added to the structure in 1893 and 1914. By our Fresher year of 1950, some 120 students were accommodated in the main block and in four temporary army huts installed in the parking area to accept the bulging enrolments of the early post-war years. Even the Freshers had their own room. In 1953 the freestanding, modern "Reid" Building was built to replace the huts, enlarging the College and greatly improving the quality of its accommodation.

The 1950s were an interesting period at the University, heavily influenced by the many ex-servicemen of the time. The prevailing ethos in college was somewhat right-wing, hearty and xenophobic. The Fresher system was prosecuted with enthusiasm and mainly in good spirit apart from the usual occasional excesses by a small minority of bullies, hardly a problem for a boarding school survivor. In 1949 the College had been recovering from significant administrative traumas which had culminated in the resignation of a former Principal. So throughout most of my time at St Andrew's we were privileged to have the Rev John McIntyre as Principal.

This formidable Scottish theologian and linguist had been Hunter-Baillie Professor of Systematic Theology and Ethics at St Andrew's Theological Hall of Sydney University since 1946 and was acting Principal in 1948. Young, handsome, and charming, he displayed an effortless gift for the firm but sympathetic leadership required in the seemingly difficult task of reconciling his youthful enthusiasm and Christian values with the sometimes conflicting agenda of his charges. Respected, almost revered by all, Dr McIntyre returned to Edinburgh in 1956 to become Professor of Divinity.

There were many medical students in college and, because they stayed longer than most, they often became prominent in student affairs.

Sports were popular and well supported and contributed greatly to the "College Spirit". Andrew's generally fared well in the Rawson Cup competition against the other university colleges in swimming, rowing, rugby, tennis, cricket and rifle shooting. From time to time more social intercollegiate contests were arranged between second VIIIs and XVs, a popular outlet for the less gifted sportsmen among us.

A significant fringe benefit of college life was our exposure to students and academics of other faculties. Suitably lubricated bull sessions extended far into the night and discourse on literature, music, theatre, life, love, theology and philosophy ameliorated somewhat the philistinism of "butchers", "greasers" [Medical and Engineering students] and the like. More organised cultural activities including revue, dramatics, debating and music were generally well-attended.

Each year a formal ball and two informals were enjoyed, and more frequent open nights provided the other officially sanctioned social activities. Partners were often recruited from The Women's College or even Sancta Sophia College, but the thousand or so student nurses living in next door at the hospital could not be overlooked.

Extramurally, The Marlborough and Grose Farm Hotels enjoyed their devoted followings. Greek cafes, especially Jim and John's in King Street and Mick's in Missenden Road, were popular courtship venues, later superseded by the novel Continental sophistication of the Astoria Coffee Lounge. Here was a suitable spot for tongue tied swains to press their courtship with tempting morsels of raisin toast and coffee.

Medical school

In 1950 the Sydney University Medical School was still recovering from the constraints of World War II. The University buildings were rundown and overfull. Admission was essentially unrestricted apart from a minor matriculation standard at the High School Leaving Certificate examinations, and former servicemen were entitled to enrolment without any restriction. As a result, classes were ridiculously large, with about 350 students in my freshman year. Not for long, though. Of our Fresher year many fell at the academic hurdles in First, Second and Third years. The examinations were an effective but very inefficient triage method which selected those with a talent for passing exams, often with minimal preparation, from the much larger number of those then "qualified" to attend University.

First year included the basic sciences of Botany, Zoology, Physics and Chemistry. Most of these subjects had been covered for most pupils in the final year of high school although Chemistry, especially Organic Chemistry, required a bit of extra work. Less than 100 of the 350 students passed the examination at the first attempt and a handful more at the deferred "Post", a repeat exam of the borderline failed subjects.

Second year included almost all new subject matter including Human Anatomy and Physiology, Biochemistry and Histology. Prof Burkitt, who taught Anatomy, was famous for falling asleep in his own lectures. Frank S Cotton had made a reputation during the war for participating in human centrifuge experiments, the scientific basis for the vital "anti-G" suit required by fighter pilots. An indifferent lecturer, his efforts were described by some as "SFA from FSC". His main interest was sports physiology and he had attracted some keen young researchers including Forbes Carlisle, an up-and-coming Olympic swimming coach, among the first to stress fitness training as distinct from technique. Sadly, Cotton was killed in a traffic accident while cycling along Parramatta Road a few years later.

Third year took the basic sciences to a higher level including Neuroanatomy and Neurophysiology. Again, these were testing examinations and the failure rate was very high. For the final term of this year the surviving students began preclinical studies in topics such as Pathology and Pharmacology and the pass rate became much more acceptable.

In fourth year, we finally tackled the basics of Clinical Medicine and Surgery as we came in contact with real live patients in the Royal Prince Alfred outpatient clinics and at the bedside. Lectures at the New Medical School in the morning were followed by Outpatients sessions and Inpatient rounds conducted by the mostly excellent honorary teachers in the course of their caring for the patients. With our smart new uniform of a short white coat denoting our lowly status we began to feel part of the great organisation of the Royal Prince Alfred Hospital. The pocket of that white coat held our magic talismans; a shiny new stethoscope and a pencil torch. A photograph of me in 1953 appears on page 37.

Fifth year was devoted to various specialties including Obstetrics and Gynaecology, surgical specialties, Dermatology, Ear Nose and Throat, Ophthalmology, Psychiatry and Public Health. Best of all from my point of view was Paediatrics. During this term our morning lectures at the Royal Alexandra Hospital for Children at Camperdown were given by the extraordinary teachers, Sir Lorimer Dods, T Y Nelson, and numerous others. Paediatrics seemed like a microcosm of Medicine and Surgery, still small enough and sufficiently coherent for a student to comprehend in the round. For the first time, everything fitted together to make sense. The children's outpatients' clinics were conducted in a Dickensian facility near Railway Square. At least it had good transport, with plentiful buses, trams and trains, and the grim, blue-tiled interior gave a semblance of cleanliness, if little warmth.

Final year was serious. Most frivolity and non-essential socialisation were kept to a minimum and almost everyone worked hard at their heavy textbooks, tutorials, and teaching rounds. The final exams were testing and we awaited the oral "viva voce" examinations with trepidation. I was well prepared, and passed well enough.

University years had not been entirely wasted; as well as the academic course, some six years in residence at St Andrew's College established a few social and sporting skills. At various times I represented the college at Debating, Rifle Shooting, in Reviews and in social intercollegiate Rowing and Rugby, and sailing was an early sporting interest outside of university.

I also participated in the first two productions of the St Andrew's College Dramatic Society, produced in a makeshift theatre in the College dining room. In Goldsmith's *She Stoops to Conquer* I played "An innkeeper", and in Bernard Shaw's *Pygmalion*, I was "Second bystander". My real contributions were in set building, backstage, and the primitive special effects of the time. One of the best applauded lines in *Pygmalion* was when Alan Kendall's Henry Higgins calls Eliza "A disgrace to the noble architecture of these columns" while the flimsy batten and hessian Covent Garden facsimiles wavered on an unsteady stage made by cramming all the dining room tables together at the far end of the room. The Dramatic Society continues to produce satisfactory plays nearly seventy years after its inception.

At the end of 1955 the St Andrew's group of Bob Oakeshott, Ian Pryde, Lindsay Roberts and I passed our exams and Bill Bevan was successful at the Deferred exam. Given that our studies had been prosecuted with varying diligence and significant distractions, we owed much to our college tutors, particularly Ron Wilde in Anatomy, Vernon Barling, Bill Costello and Bruce Pearson in Surgery, Jim Isbister and Bruce Smith in Medicine and John Knox in Gynaecology.

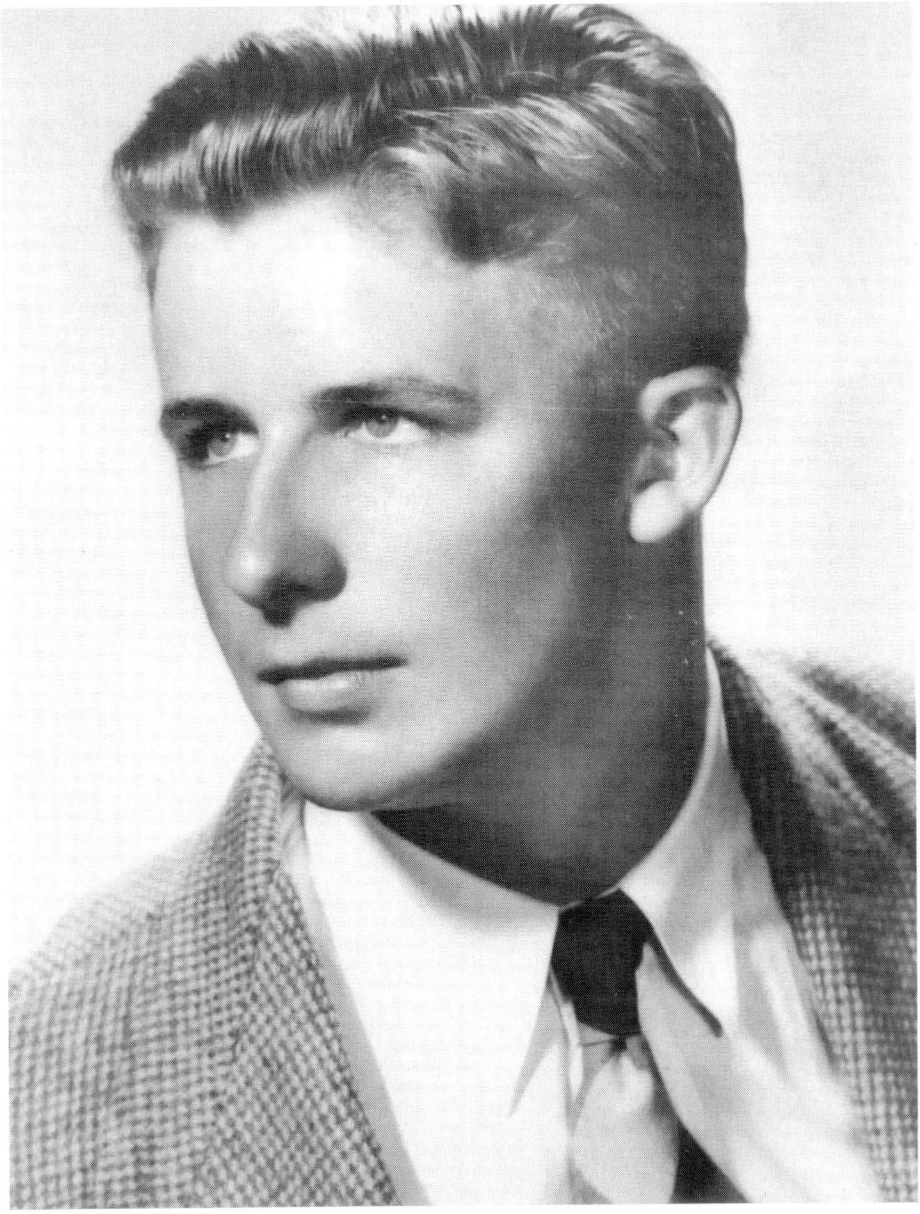

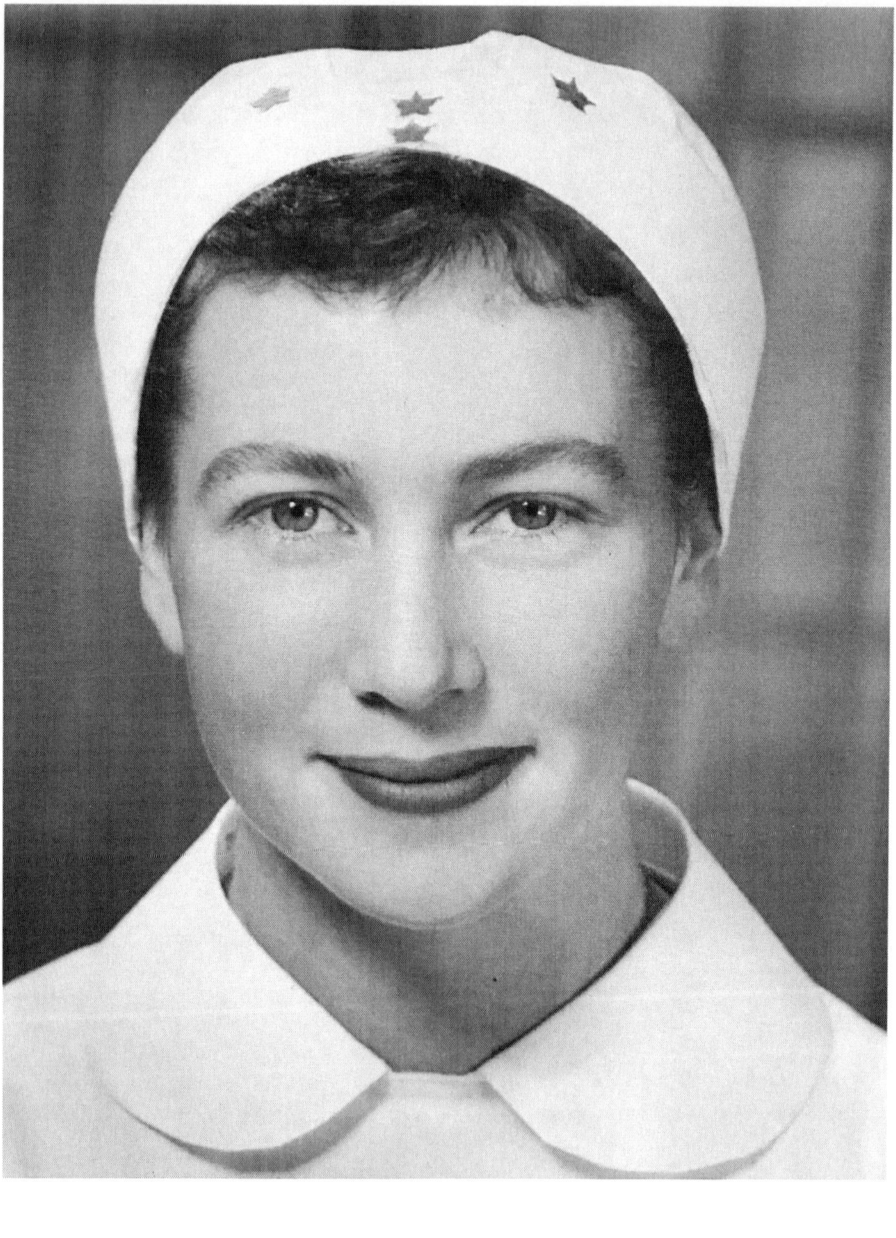

Chapter 3: Royal Prince Alfred Hospital years

By 22 years of age, I was at last grown up and it was time to put away childish things. Armed with my brand-new qualification of Bachelor of Medicine and Bachelor of Surgery from the Sydney University Medical School, reasonably equipped with the theoretical knowledge of the day, almost completely innocent of practical skills, clad in short white coat, long white trousers and white shoes, I joined my equally green fellow neophytes at the Royal Prince Alfred Hospital as a Junior Resident Medical Officer (now called an Intern).

Junior Resident Medical Officer

I had not had a stellar early undergraduate career but became seriously engaged in studying hard for the clinical years of Medical School and got a reasonably good pass in the final examination. It was a privilege to be selected as JRMO at Prince Alfred and I made the most of it.

JRMOs lived in the hospital, two or three to a room at that time. Rosters were either one-in-two nights or one-in-three nights on duty, in addition to the normal working day of eight o'clock in the morning to six o'clock in the evening. On the night off, as soon as all work was completed after six, it was permissible to leave the hospital but everyone had to return by one o'clock in the morning and make a Ward round before going to sleep. This was a demanding schedule but most of us were keen and conscientious and got on with the job.

Internship is an extraordinary learning experience as a huge bank of theoretical knowledge is brought to bear on practical patient management and integration with hospital systems and culture.

The Junior Resident Medical Officer was the lowest form of medical life in a hospital. He (occasionally she in those days) was the clerk who wrote the medical histories and organised tests, further treatments and procedures for patients. He was general dogsbody, at everyone else's beck and call. His was the responsibility for any errors or misfortunes; he was indeed at the bottom of the pile. He was assigned to a team or ward for terms of about 10 weeks. If he was smart he worked hard, said little, paid attention, and learned all he could from his seniors and especially from the head Sister of the ward. These Ward Sisters were key to the continuity of ward management.

Many were former Military Nurses, often legendary battle-axes, and could and did rule their juniors, especially the trainee nurses, with an iron hand. But they were usually very knowledgeable and competent in their sphere. They offered a fund of practical knowhow about their ward, the patients, and how to get things done.

The terms that I particularly remember include Gynaecology, Surgery, Medicine, Casualty (usually called Emergency these days), a relieving term, and Urology.

First was the Gynaecology team of Malcolm Stening, Margaret Mulvey, and Britnell Fraser. George and Malcolm Stening were fine technicians and this was my first taste of systematised surgery, by which I mean standardised procedures carried out consistently and efficiently without hurry, but also without wasted time or movement.

For General Surgery I worked for Alexander Skeffington Johnson and his Junior, John Spence. Johnson was a very popular and decent man, exceedingly conscientious, almost querulous. Standard abdominal operations went well. Frequent operations included gastrectomies for peptic ulcer disease and hemicolectomies for carcinoma of the colon [This refers to removal or "resection" of large portions of the stomach or large bowel]. Alex was a good cautious operator and his patients did well. His Junior colleague, Jack Spence was a large, loud, attractive man who had made his reputation as a battlefield surgeon. His speed and decisiveness did not serve so well in civilian practice and the postoperative course was sometimes prolonged and complicated.

Tom Greenaway was my boss in General Medicine. Tom was tall, articulate, impeccably dressed and impossibly knowledgeable. This was a golden age for physicians at Prince Alfred and Greenaway, along with Bill Morrow, John Kempson Maddox, Billy Bye, and the following generation of Ruthven Blackburn, Stan Goulston and others were leaders in Australia at the time. Indeed, it was the final flowering of the Generalists, theoretically competent in all areas of medical diagnosis and treatment, as the reality of specialisation and fragmentation began to take hold. Tom Greenaway's registrar at the time was his son, John, later to become a distinguished specialist in his own right. As well as the general run of medical problems we frequently had patients with rare and interesting conditions, as Greenaway was a highly reputable expert in these fields.

In the afternoons, in addition to our normal ward duties, we were assigned to give anaesthetics in the Anderson Stewart Theatres. Ivor Hotten was the bombastic head of Anaesthesia. More influential from my point of view was Bruce Clifton, recently returned from a stint with the British Commonwealth Occupation Force in Japan, and an outstanding teacher. Anaesthesia was enjoyable, with its combination of technical skills and pharmacological, medical and surgical knowledge. In particular, the insights into physiology stood me in good stead later.

The relieving term was just that. One of my duties was a short spell as Blood Bank Resident. This was largely a technician's job involving cross matching
of blood, supplying it as required to the operating theatres and wards, and setting up elective transfusions. Useful skills, significant responsibility because of the risk of catastrophic blood mismatches, but not very challenging.

Urology was a nicely circumscribed surgical specialty, and the surgeons at Prince Alfred were likeable and competent. Malcolm Earlam was particularly skilful, and Angus Walker-Smith supportive and friendly. For most of this term I acted in effect as Registrar, a post usually occupied by an advanced trainee surgeon, because Dennis Arnold, who had been appointed Fellow in Urology, had not yet returned from England. This was one of several occasions in which I was serendipitously promoted above my true level of seniority, and they were very productive learning experiences.

Casualty, or Emergency, was testing, as we junior doctors were thrown in at the deep end to care for whatever patients came along. Traffic accidents, broken bones, acute illnesses of every kind, some drunks, some mentally ill and some malingerers, all took their chances with us. There was still a lot of light industry in the inner suburbs of Sydney so we saw many industrial accidents such as hand and eye injuries and foreign bodies. We could call on others one or two years our senior but were generally expected to sort out the problems, admit those patients who needed it, and send the others away with reassurance and medication of variable effectiveness. Fortunately, the default setting is that most illnesses cure themselves without much help. It was a far cry from the hand holding which junior doctors "enjoy" today in the Emergency Departments.

1957

1957 was an extraordinary year, as I became a Senior Resident Medical Officer and, resplendent in my new uniform of a real doctor's long white coat, undertook more responsibilities.

The story of Marilyn's and my marriage really starts in mid 1953, when I had left it perilously late to try to find a partner for one of our college informal balls. Fate delivered me to a regular teaching session at the dingy Brown Street Surgical Outpatient Department at Prince Alfred where I noted our bustling nurse, Marilyn McKenzie, in her neatly starched white pinafore. Having thoughtfully sneaked a look at her name badge, I later phoned the Nurses' Home at the hospital and haltingly asked her out for coffee. Notwithstanding my inarticulate attempts at conversation, she agreed to accompany me to the Ball. We didn't have much to say there either, but there must have been some attraction because, after I had returned from my winter vacation, we met again. It became something of an evening routine to go to Jim and John's Greek Cafe, on King Street, Newtown, sometimes by ourselves, sometimes in company with one or more other couples for coffee and toast.

Later I was invited for a weekend at Gosford to meet Marilyn's parents. Whenever we had days off, that became our courtship. A bit later, she also came to holiday with my family at Nymboida. A photograph of Marilyn in 1956 appears on page 38. After we had both graduated, in early 1956, we became engaged.

In February 1957 we were married at St Stephen's Church in Macquarie Street. The wedding party was minute, just our immediate families and a few friends, while the church was the largest Presbyterian Kirk in the town. After a motoring honeymoon which took us through Melbourne to the Great Ocean Road, we were lucky to find a small apartment which had just become available in Haberfield. In the few months we lived there we settled into a pattern of long working hours, frequent nights on duty, and somehow learning the civilities of married life. We also had a couple of excellent parties with our friends, nearly all of them my contemporary young doctors and their wives and girlfriends.

Soon we had moved to a bigger, better lodging in the lower floor of a duplex apartment at Balgowlah, where we stayed until 1963. By November 1957 I was working all the hours there were as part of the open-heart surgery team and Marilyn was nearing the end of her pregnancy. John was born on 5th December, and I had little time to spend with either of them.

Back to the beginning of 1957: my first term was Obstetrics, an interesting field with many practical things to learn and do. The outstanding senior Obstetrician at King George V hospital was the articulate and elegant Professor Bruce Mayes. Also noteworthy as teachers were Clinical Superintendent Rodney Shearman and Registrar Alan Bradfield. Bradfield was especially impressive with his suavely handsome, well-groomed manner, his kind and considerate dealings with everyone, especially the patients, and his biting wit in private.

Second term was a General Surgical one with Dr Fred Neische. Old Fred was a much admired surgeon and a very competent one, but very old-school and unbending. His Junior Surgeon was Frank Mills, about whom I will write much more during this memoir. Frank was the most senior of the Junior Surgeons at Prince Alfred, approaching his late forties. He had performed the first mitral valve operations in Sydney, and also the first Blalock shunts for tetralogy of Fallot.

[Mitral stenosis was a narrowing of the mitral valve which partially obstructed blood flow from the left atrium to the left ventricle. The narrowing resulted from inflammation and scarring due to rheumatic fever. The operation consisted of reopening the valve using an index finger introduced through the left atrium, sometimes supplemented by various instruments, while the heart continued beating.

[The tetralogy of Fallot was a congenital heart defect in which babies were born with a large opening between the right and left ventricle or pumping chambers, plus a severe narrowing of the outflow part of the heart leading to the lungs. Blue venous blood was diverted away from the lungs into the aorta, reducing the uptake of oxygen and causing persisting cyanosis – the "blue baby" syndrome. Blalock's operation consisted of increasing pulmonary blood flow by sewing a subclavian artery which normally would supply an arm onto the pulmonary artery, so increasing the blood flow to the lungs.]

Mills was a small, intense man, highly intelligent, and inclined to be taciturn. He was one of the few surgeons in those days who was interested in experimental surgery in the animal laboratory.

At the time I joined his team, Frank was beginning to prepare for open heart surgery using a pump oxygenator. Each Friday morning, we took a handful of instruments to the lab, set up our apparatus and went through the complex sequence of connecting our animal to the machine, bypassing the heart and lungs, then resuming normal circulation if we could. Hard work the first couple of hundred tries! Frank Mills and I were bonded in adversity through these trials. I return to this topic in "Pioneer Open Heart Surgery" below.

Another great technician for whom I worked several times during my training was Joe McMahon. Joe boasted of being a disciple of Sir Alexander McCormack and Sir John McKelvie and had a palette of operations which he performed with extraordinary fluency. Though temperamentally a bit of a bully, he was usually satisfied with perfection. He knew what had to be done, he knew what he expected of his trainees, and provided they supplied it unfailingly, he was easy enough to get on with.

The Page Chest Pavilion had been opened in the second half of 1957. It was one of a series of chest hospitals funded by the Australian Government for the treatment of pulmonary tuberculosis. During its planning Sir Herbert Schlinck, Chairman of the Board of Directors of the hospital, had arranged for additional floors to be added, originally planned for nurses' accommodation but subsequently revised to become additional wards for non-tuberculous patients.

Following Tom Fraser, I became the second Resident Medical Officer in Thoracic Medicine in the Page Chest Pavilion, an excellent term with an outstanding group of physicians and teachers. Drs Cotter Harvey and Maurice Joseph were Senior Chest Physicians and Peter Harvey, Cotter's son, was simultaneously serving as Clinical Superintendent of the new hospital and as a Junior Chest Physician; another superb teacher. This chest unit functioned very well, providing busy medical outpatient clinics, bronchoscopy clinics, and inpatient care. Joint medical and surgical conferences were an excellent introduction to Thoracic Surgery, and helping Peter Harvey to commission a new Hospital was very stimulating.

Lung cancer was a common problem. Tuberculosis was coming under control with streptomycin and the other new antimicrobial treatments but several patients with residual lung cavities required intricate resections of the lung. There were also many remaining cases of suppurative lung disease following a pandemic of antibiotic resistant staphylococcus in the previous year or two.

Earlier that year, the Clinical Superintendent, Dr Bob Packard, had assigned me to care for a patient with tetanus, for whom he was trialling a new regimen of treatment. Tetanus, known from the time of Hippocrates as a killer, had traditionally been treated as an infectious disease in the Isolation Ward, a cottage remote from the main hospital buildings. This was not ideal because the patients experiencing the severe muscle spasms caused by tetanus toxin suffered respiratory insufficiency, and often required urgent tracheostomy. Specialised medical, surgical and nursing skills were lacking on site. Results were poor and mortality remained high.

Packard reasoned that combination therapy using the benzodiazepine sedative chlorpromazine and the long-acting barbiturate Amytal might better control the spasms. More importantly, he recognised the need to care for these critically ill patients in the main hospital and allocated a single room attached to one of the medical wards for that purpose. A "special" nurse was allocated to care solely for that patient round-the-clock and I was to be the dedicated medical officer.

Our first patient was a teenaged girl who was sedated for about 10 days, and she made a full recovery. No doubt this did my reputation no harm. Packard and I reported this treatment in *The Medical Journal of Australia*; my first scientific publication. [Soon afterward, this therapy was superseded by full anaesthesia, muscle relaxation with curare, and supporting the patient with a mechanical ventilator until they had fully recovered, a more controlled treatment.]

I imagine that it was my collaboration with Bob Packard, along with my experimental laboratory work with Mills, that led to my being appointed as the Surgical Registrar to the Open Heart project which was to occur at the end of 1957 (see Pioneer Open Heart Surgery below).

Maybe Dr Packard had confidence in my general competence and common sense and, although very junior for such a task, I was as well versed in the new technology as anybody else at that time. Maybe nobody else wanted the job.

I will devote separate sections of this memoir firstly to a brief history of open heart surgery to that time, and secondly to that memorable visit in which Drs Bahnson and Spencer introduced the technique to Royal Prince Alfred Hospital and New South Wales.

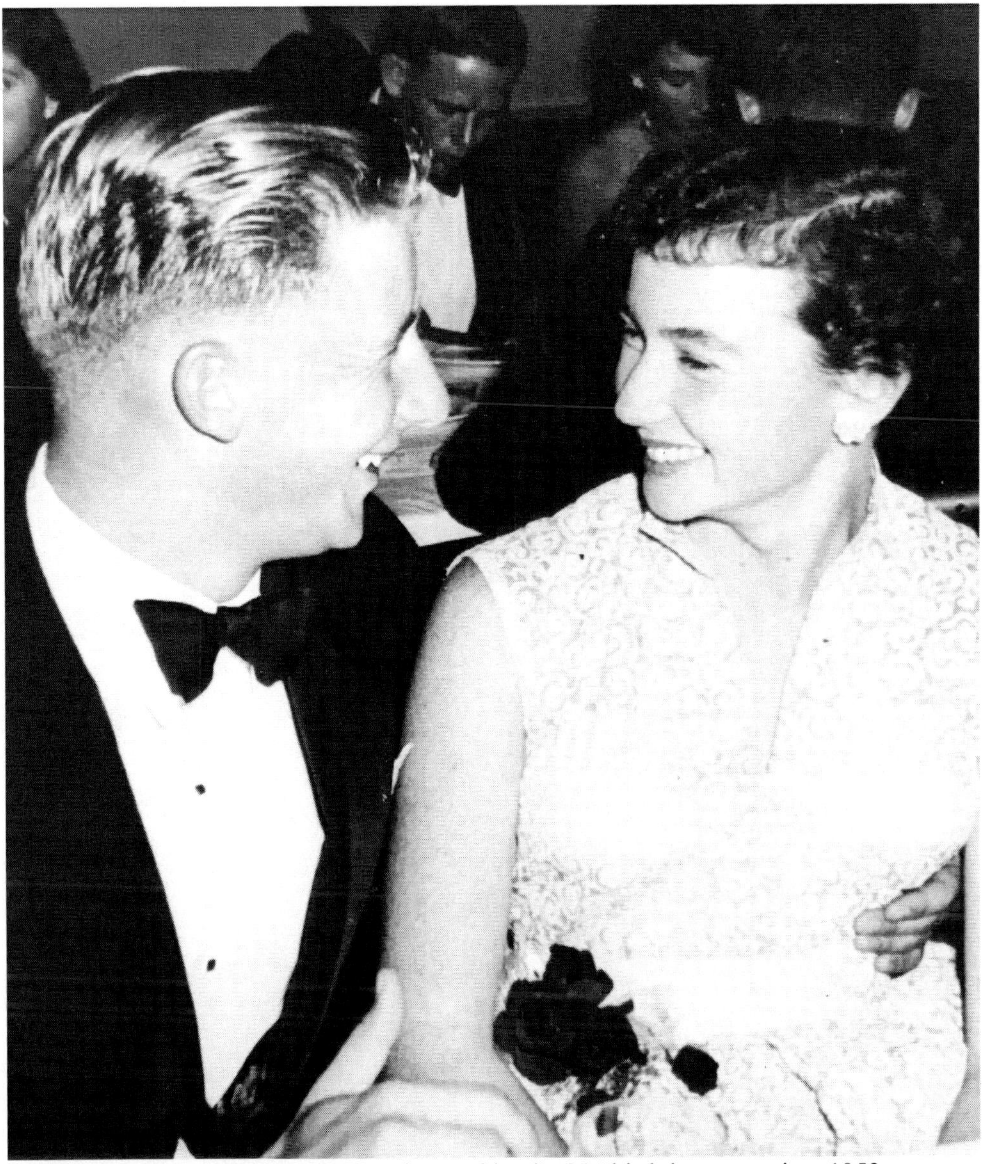

Tim Cartmill and Marilyn McKenzie at a friend's 21st birthday party circa 1953

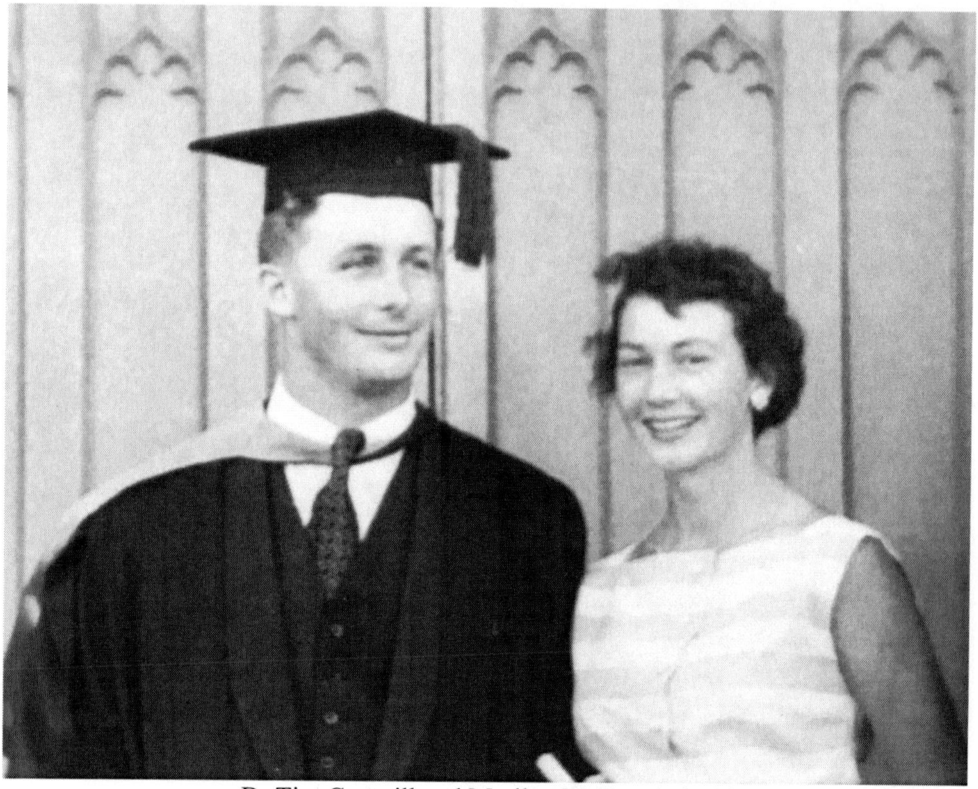

Dr Tim Cartmill and Marilyn McKenzie in 1956

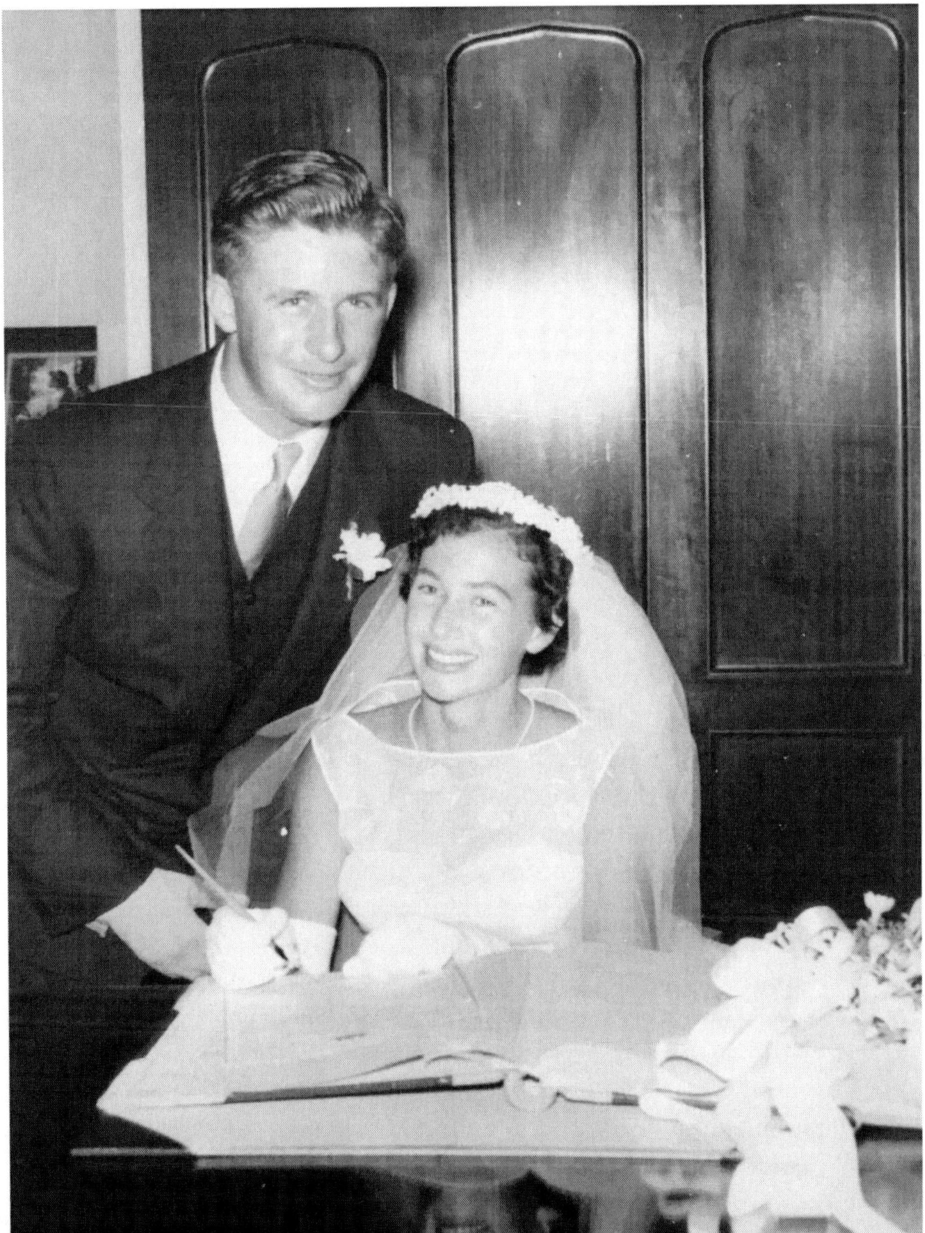

Tim and Marilyn Cartmill in 1957

1958

In 1958 I became the first Registrar in Thoracic Surgery at the new Page Chest Pavilion of the Royal Prince Alfred Hospital. This was a very stimulating and enjoyable period professionally. The new program in open-heart surgery slowly gathered momentum although we had only one operating day per week to begin with because of the tremendous logistic challenges. Ten units of fresh blood were routinely cross matched for each operation. The pump oxygenator had to be thoroughly washed, then gas-sterilised overnight, and we were years away from working out the practicalities of full-time postoperative care.

Cardiac Surgery staff remained as in 1957, that is Rowan Nicks, Alexander (Sandy) Grant, Frank Mills, and Paul Tomlinson. In turn, one of them would operate and another act as first assistant. A much better arrangement would have been to have only two surgeons, assisting one another time and time about until the caseload became much greater. We were much better served in Anaesthesia. Bruce Clifton was Anaesthetist while Jeanne Collison operated the heart-lung machine. Bob Pragnell, a recruit from the laboratory technician staff, was our perfectionist Pump Technician and remained so for many years.

Cardiology also took some time to function properly in the new hospital. Senior cardiologists John Kempson Maddox and John Halliday were part-time Honorary Physicians, expert by the standards of the day. Ted Halliday and Dr John (Dick) Richards were junior cardiologists, Dick having recently returned from postgraduate study in London. The Medical Director of the Hallstrom Institute of Cardiology, Dr Bruce Sinclair-Smith, was a salaried staff member and full-time Physician to the Institute. Louis Bernstein was Registrar in Cardiology and became my friend, ally and invaluable colleague.

As well as Cardiac Surgery, the new hospital now housed the Thoracic Surgery unit. Rowan Nicks had been appointed the first Staff Surgeon to the Page Chest Pavilion. John (Joe) McMahon was senior Thoracic Surgeon, along with his duties as Honorary General Surgeon to the hospital. Sandy Grant was a Junior Honorary Surgeon at that time. Between them they provided all the lung surgery services and most of the oesophageal surgery as well.

Primary Fellowship

Concurrently with my clinical work in 1958, the third year after I graduated, I decided to "have a go" at sitting the Primary examination for Fellowship of the Royal Australasian College of Surgeons. In this I was largely influenced by David Glenn, one year my senior, who had achieved the same thing the previous year.

This Primary was a difficult examination, one that most candidates failed at the first attempt. The subjects were broad and complex. Anatomy was examined at the highest level and caused the most casualties. Physiology and Pathology seemed easier but were no pushover. I worked really hard but it was a very busy year and, with hindsight, I should have taken it more seriously. I do not advocate a half-hearted approach to examinations or any serious task. If it's worth doing it is worth trying to overwhelm at the first attempt rather than just seeing what turns up.

In short, I failed the exam. Almost immediately, I applied for a half-time job as Demonstrator at the Sydney University Medical School Anatomy Department, headed by Prof Norman "Black Mac" Macintosh. I was one of a small group selected for that position in 1959 and it was a huge advantage. Macintosh himself contributed little after selecting the Demonstrators but his Senior Lecturer, Cedric Thwaites, was an outstanding teacher and gave us every attention. Before the academic year started and the students appeared, each of us had about a month in which to fully dissect a cadaver, a rare privilege. Although each of us worked solo we also spent our time together examining the subject in the finest detail and were constantly grilled by Thwaites to develop our viva voce technique. Then, as the students did their own dissection at a much slower pace, we spent part of every day in the dissection room working with them, talking and living Anatomy. There is no substitute for such intensive exposure.

At the same time, we were studying all the other material in Physiology and Pathology and polishing our presentation skills. Small wonder that, at the end of the year, all except one of our group of eight demonstrators passed the Primary exam. The one failure had been by far the least diligent of the group, though he finally succeeded and became a Radiologist. One of my colleagues became an outstanding Obstetrics and Gynaecology specialist and the rest of us all succeeded in various surgical specialties.

At the same time as teaching at the Department of Anatomy, I spent half my time in 1959 as Registrar in Thoracic Surgery. Among other things I operated the heart-lung machine during the heart procedures, and cared for the patients post operatively.

Best of all, our daughter Alison was born in 1959 and we had settled in to the crazy routine of a young doctor. I was working and studying for most of that time and Marilyn was busy caring for the children and the household. This was to be our routine until we left in 1963 for America.

1960

Having passed the Primary examination of the Fellowship of the Royal Australasian College of Surgeons at the end of 1959, I became Registrar in General Surgery at Prince Alfred the following year. This was a period of hard and increasingly responsible work in the wards and operating theatres, supervising junior medical staff, arranging consultations, taking care of emergencies, mastering increasingly complex procedures, and at the same time studying intensely in preparation for the Final exam.

Some important mentors during this year included Norman Wyndham, Vernon Barling, and Frank Mills.

Norman Wyndham was a complex character, genuinely religious, with a supercilious manner that he used to camouflage his shyness. He was a genuine scholar, who spoke at least a few words of many languages. Once, when we were students, as our group clustered around a patient's bed, Norm impressed us mightily by conversing with the man in his native German tongue. As we filed away, the patient detained one of our number and asked him quietly: “Hey, mate, what was that all about?"

Because of his affinity for the transcendental, he was often surreptitiously called God. As usual, this was not the best kept secret. During one abdominal operation, when he noticed a tired assistant inadvertently putting too much tension on a newly sewn anastomosis joining two sections of bowel he intoned: “Whom God has brought together, let no man put asunder!” On another occasion he went to scrub his hands at the row of basins in the old Anderson-Stewart operating theatres at Prince Alfred, standing beside Fred Neische. Fred, rather deaf, exclaimed: “Oh, Norman, I did not hear you arrive!” Replied Norm: "Did you not hear the trumpets?" He was also a well-intentioned teacher with a wealth of knowledge and I found him good fun to engage with intellectually.

Wyndham's Junior Surgeon at that time was Vernon Barling, a very different man, open and generous. He lived for teaching, and believed that simple ways were often best, at least until one mastered the fundamentals. So he stuck to the textbook, in this case Hamilton Bailey, and followed it to the letter. Any reasonably intelligent trainee could soon do most things competently, provided he was not too clumsy. A favourite expression when trouble loomed was: “At moments like these you need Minties!” Perhaps not surprisingly, Barling was also quick to increase the responsibilities which he was prepared to thrust on young people. We were greatly distressed when he died just a few years later in a motor accident.

Frank Mills had now become a Senior Surgeon, and an exacting teacher. He was a meticulous technician and a demanding task master. When one had gained his confidence he extended a lot of trust.

Frank had uncanny clinical judgment, and often pulled a rabbit out of the hat by ordering the test no one else had thought of, or by producing a technical trick he had picked up somewhere around the world.

In addition to full-time clinical work and book learning, I participated in an intensive course organised by the College of Surgeons and run by a group of dedicated surgeons of the Sydney teaching hospitals. This course comprised both lectures and clinical demonstrations in preparation for the final Fellowship exams. The course brought together an excellent group of participants, including some from interstate. It was personally and professionally enjoyable, and contributed to our success in the examination.

The Final Examinations included several written papers and extensive viva voce exams. These vivas included a long case, in which each candidate was allotted a patient from whom they had to elicit and write a full history and perform a clinical examination, and then submit to close interrogation by a pair of examiners. Short cases involved rapid examination of a series of diverse patients, essentially requiring a spot diagnosis (that is giving a diagnosis after a brief examination, or even on sight). Particular credit seemed to be earned for seeing as many patients as possible in the allotted time. The marking system was a sudden-death one; any significant error at any stage was rewarded by failure.

The announcement of exam results was a tense time. On the evening of the final exam all the candidates assembled outside the headquarters of the Royal Australian College of Physicians in Macquarie Street, to be summoned one by one by the College Secretary to enter the front hall. Each candidate would either be invited to walk upstairs to join the examiners for celebratory sherry, or,
if unsuccessful, cast back into the darkness of the street. I was one of the happy sherry sippers.

Completion of formal training in Surgery is a great personal milestone. It carries considerable kudos in the medical profession and recognition in the broader society. It opens the door to the next phase, really to a lifetime of gathering and sharing proficiency, knowledge, experience, judgement and reputation. The first door that opened for me was an offer to participate in a period of dedicated research with Frank Mills.

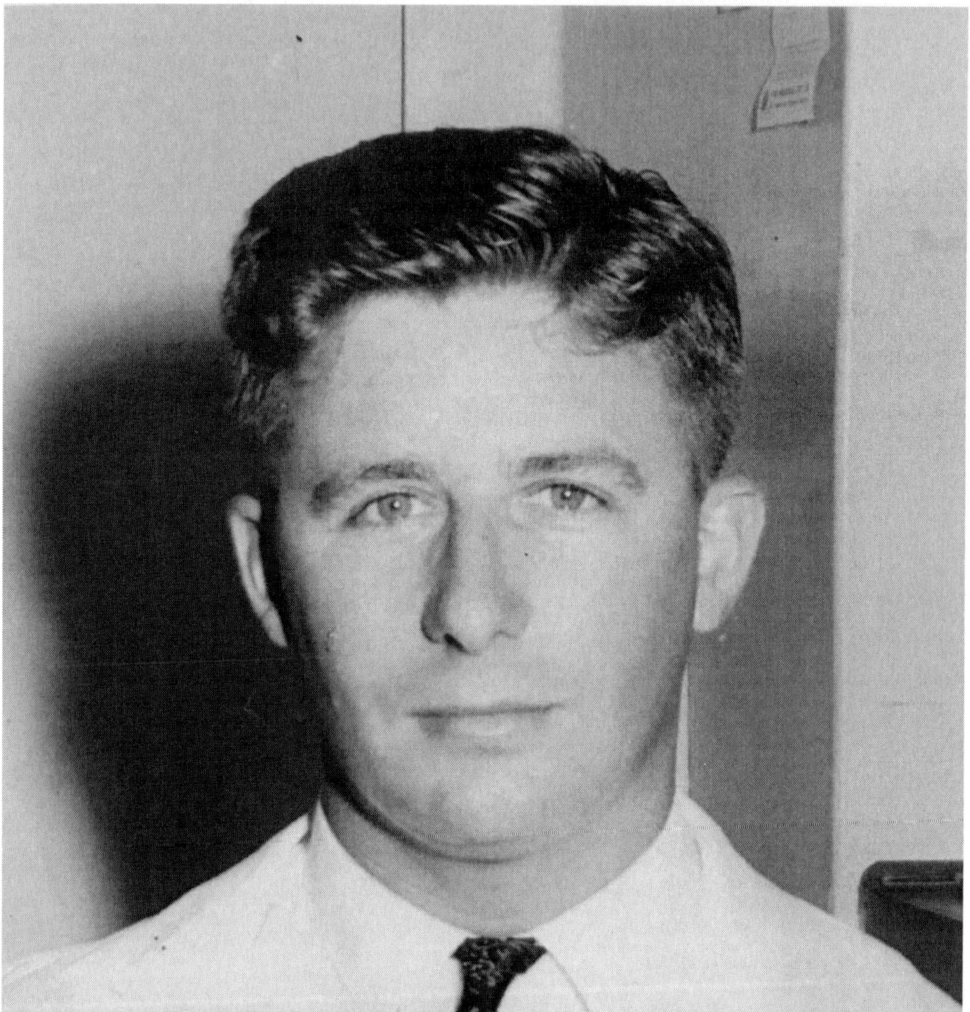

Tim as a Registrar in 1957

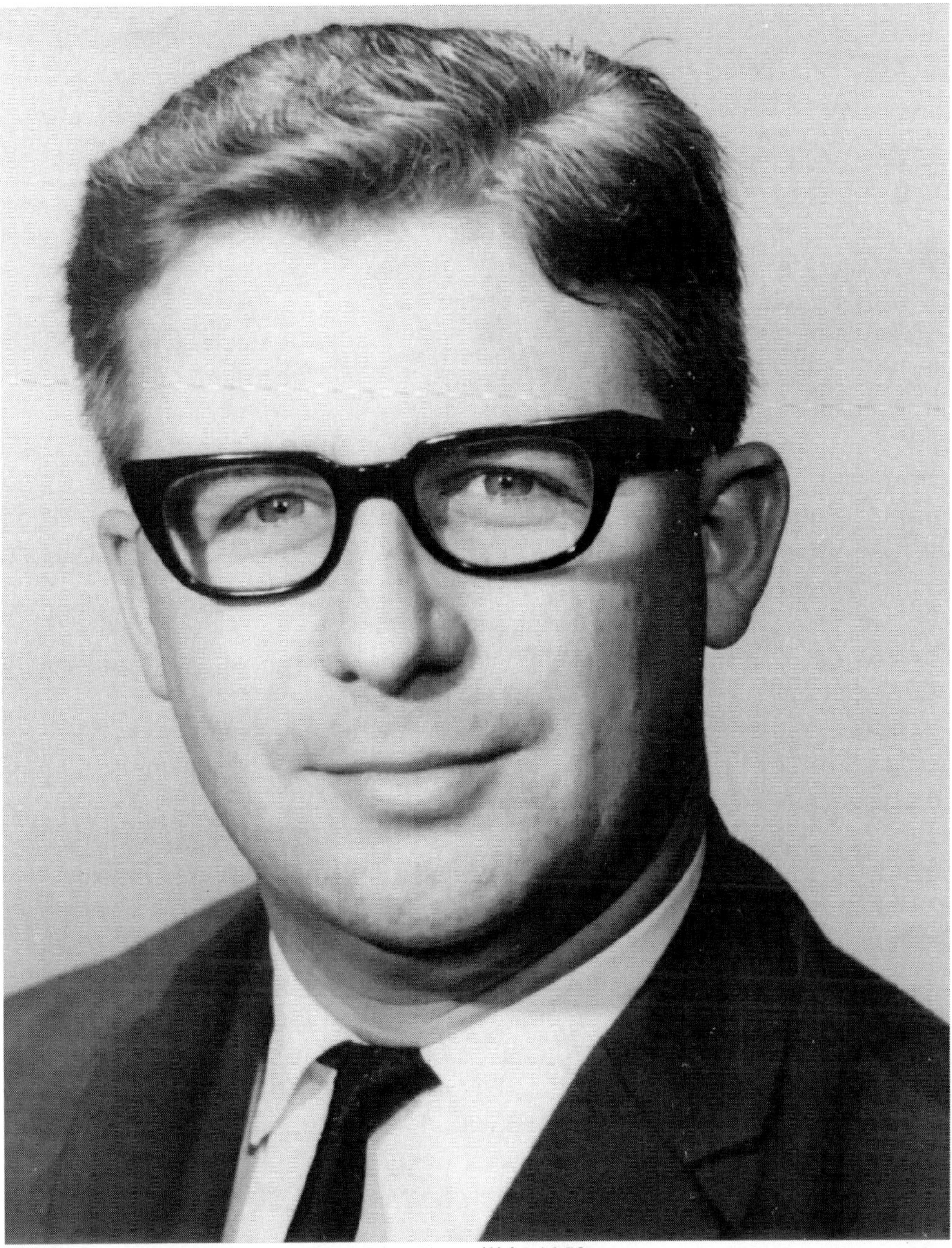

Tim Cartmill in 1959

Chemotheraphy Research

After I had passed my FRACS examination, Frank Mills asked me to join him in a research project funded by the NSW Cancer Council. Ever a restless intelligence, he had become interested in the new field of Regional Chemotherapy which was beginning to develop overseas, particularly at the MD Anderson Institute in Houston, Texas.

Chemotherapy relies on the principle that metabolically active cancer tissues or cells will be destroyed by certain toxic chemotherapeutic agents. Unfortunately, these drugs are also highly toxic to other actively growing cells, particularly those of the blood and bone marrow. It was hoped that refined surgical techniques could deliver the drugs selectively in higher concentrations to the local area required, while the remainder of the body might be spared some of the toxic side effects. Hence the term Regional Chemotherapy.

We investigated two main techniques: intra-arterial infusion, and regional perfusion using a small heart-lung machine or pump-oxygenator (see below for explanation).

John Loewenthal, Professor of Surgery at Sydney University, agreed to host our program in his department. Our plan was to develop the techniques and equipment in the animal laboratory at the Medical School and apply the methods for patients under Frank Mills' care at RPAH.

First we assembled our special equipment. For the arterial infusions we purchased a special miniaturised DeBakey style roller pump capable of delivering a small volume of dilute methotrexate solution over a period of several days. Later, one of our technicians, Bob Ellis, manufactured a local version of this pump, using a more precise stepping motor. These pumps compressed a small diameter silicone rubber tube using a small roller, and proved satisfactory. For the regional perfusions we purchased a heart-lung machine from Ebs-Ray pumps at Brookvale who supplied the pump chassis and one of their smallest Kay-Cross style oxygenators.

We employed a technician to care for our equipment and take care of the animals.

Techniques

Intra-arterial infusion relied on placing a fine catheter (tube) in the arterial system to deliver Methotrexate selectively into the target area to be treated. Inserting the catheter in the correct place depended on a detailed understanding of arterial anatomy. I developed a technique to confirm the location by injecting a blue dye, Evans Blue, or later Cardio-Green, to stain the target area. We mainly used the method to treat unresectable (unremovable) cancers in areas of the head and neck, such as the tongue or mandible. As the drug was infused over several days the patients almost all improved, with the tumours shrinking and often delivering striking pain relief. It was not realistic to expect long-term cure.

Regional perfusion was technically much more complicated. The principle was to isolate the arteries and veins of a region of the body as completely as possible and then maintain its circulation by pumping blood through that area for a period of a few hours at most. The chemotherapeutic drug could be given at high dose and there was evidence that its effect could be further enhanced by raising the local temperature and also increasing the oxygen content of the blood above normal, both easily managed with a pump oxygenator. This technique was best suited for an arm or a leg, where the limb circulation could be isolated using a tourniquet. We also hoped to use it for the fore-quarter in cases of breast cancer, the idea being that the draining lymph nodes in the axilla (armpit) could be treated in preparation for breast resection. Unfortunately, it proved impractical to adequately isolate the circulation in that area of the body.

In summary, the perfusion method was of limited success. After my departure, Fred Stephens took up the infusion technique and continued to use it for many years, mostly for selected cases of liver cancer. In various guises it is still used.

We had not found "the cure for cancer" but I had the privilege of spending two and half years in an academic department, with time to read all the literature about cancer treatment and heart surgery.

I made the most of my free access to the animal laboratory, polished my skills in vascular surgery and continued to participate each week in the cardiac surgery experiments in the animal laboratory. The main impetus for this cardiac work came from Rowan Nicks who was always enthusiastic for lab work of all sorts.

In cardiac surgery our emphasis was in refining the technical aspects of cannulation, management of the equipment, and general teamwork. It was more a technical drill than a scientific endeavour. By actively participating in this practical work in a less demanding environment than clinical surgery on human patients, I quickly achieved a level of technical competence and proficiency above my real level of experience.

In summary, during my two and a half years in this combined laboratory and clinical project, I worked hard on my technique while enjoying the intellectual stimulation of the Department of Surgery, gained the growing confidence of my mentors, Frank Mills and Rowan Nicks, and capitalised on the advantage of concentrated academic study of the specialised fields of cancer chemotherapy and cardiac surgery.

The specialty of cardiac surgery was steadily gaining in success and public support, and I became convinced that I should go abroad for further training. To this end, Nicks had corresponded with his friends Owen Clagett at Mayo Clinic and Mike DeBakey in Houston. Clagett responded first and offered me a Fellowship at Mayo but because of the way in which the medical year starts in the middle of a calendar year in the United States it proved expedient to accept DeBakey's offer first. Meanwhile I had successfully applied for a Fulbright Scholarship which provided travel expenses for me and my family.

Chapter 4: The American years

It was always inevitable, given my ambitions, that I should have wanted to train in the United States, because that was where most of the cardiac surgery action was occurring at that time.

Most Australian medicos who studied abroad in those days went by ship to England. The jet aircraft such as the Boeing 707 and Douglas DC8 were brand new, and the greatly increased capacity meant that many travel companies were offering special deals. Marilyn and I chose Air France, largely because it offered a couple of nights of free accommodation in Tahiti.

We were ambitious, arrogant, naïve and poor, having scraped together a few hundred Pounds, representing all the spare cash I had in the world. Our plan was to fly with John and Alison, aged five and three, to the US West Coast, to purchase a cheap and hopefully reliable car and drive to Houston. Neither of us had been much further afield than Brisbane or Melbourne, and Australia of 1963 was a much simpler place than it is now. Among the pleasures of our trip would be the expected exposure to other cultures, customs, foods and societies. This expectation was certainly fulfilled in Tahiti, our first stop over. Greeted at the gangway by ukelele music and floral leis, accommodated in a beachside palm-thatch bure, or hut, enchanted by the night perfume of tiara Tahiti flowers, lulled by the rustling palm leaves, we slept deeply. Morning brought a marvellous French breakfast of crispy rolls and café au lait. This was the real thing, after the half-baked dreams engendered by high school French studies. Lunch consisted of a dish I remember vividly to this day: papaya au shrimp, a delectable salad of tiny shrimps in a spicy mayonnaise, served in the half papaya. Our sophistication was growing by the minute!

Dinner was served to the accompaniment of native dancing, performed by truly attractive but not totally authentic young ladies wearing short grass skirts, suspicious looking tops made of half coconut shells, and flashing pearly uniform smiles. We later learned that the Marlon Brando movie, *Mutiny on the Bounty*, had recently been filmed on these islands. To obtain the authentic

Island appearance, all the local extras had their carious teeth extracted and replaced with fine synthetic choppers.

No slouch when it came to haute cuisine, I ordered frogs legs from the menu. They tasted pretty good, especially when accompanied by heroic doses of garlic. I was somewhat nonplussed when, in the midst of chewing one of those morsels, I was dragged to the dance floor by one of those dusky beauties. Dancing has never been my forte, and my attempts to perform some cool steps, in close proximity to the jiggling coconut shells, trying to smile with a mouth full of frog's pelvis which I could neither swallow nor spit out, overreached my terpsichorian limits.

Two days later we flew to San Francisco after changing planes in Los Angeles. The great American adventure began. Even then, one needed spare change to buy all kinds of things from vending machines. I put a dollar bill into a money-changing machine at the airport and was humbled to lose it. Some witnesses allege that I kicked the apparatus. I have noticed over the years that one thing that sets the traveller off as a foreign dill is their lack of expertise with local currency. It also took us very little time to learn that everything associated with airports was at least twice as expensive as everywhere else. In a similar vein, we soon learned not to eat in hotel dining rooms but to head to the nearest drugstore.

The American drugstore was and is an extraordinary institution and I have not come across anything quite like it anywhere else. Certainly it acts as a pharmacy, but it also has an excellent cafe counter providing simple meals for very little money. Staples included bacon and eggs, ham, and hash brown potato, soggy white toast and apple jelly. There I saw for the first time a young soldier demolish a stack of a dozen pancakes doused in maple syrup. And we encountered the marvellous American institution known as the bottomless cup of coffee. For five cents in those days you could keep drinking bitter coffee till you could stand no more.

It was time to buy a car and set off on the long drive, seeing as many sites as we could on the way. For US$300, maybe equivalent to about AU150pounds, I got a seven year old Ford Mercury, the last of the side-valve V8s. With care, we thought it would take us as far as we needed to go, and so it did. We set off across the Bay and had a quick look in the Sequoia and Yosemite National Parks. It had always been part of our plan to see as many of those natural wonders as we could and their memory remains vivid. Our track to Los Angeles took us inland through the agricultural districts of the irrigated San Joaquin valley.

A contact in Los Angeles kindly arranged for us to visit Disneyland. No doubt the children enjoyed it, and it is an experience that everyone must have once in a lifetime. My overwhelming memory is the sickly sweet smell of the soft drinks and fairy floss. Soon it was time to set out across the desert. We had chosen to drive through the night to avoid the heat.

Sometime in the small hours we came to Las Vegas, and stopped for a snack. I put my few cents of change in the slot machine and predictably lost the whole lot in no time. Dawn found us somewhere in the desert in Utah. The traffic authorities here had painted an aeroplane symbol on the highway at one-mile intervals so that their spy in the sky could time cars and detect speeding from on high.

We tried to find the cheapest available motel and were happy to enjoy a swimming pool if it had one. The cooling system was a large fan in the window. Dinner consisted of soggy hamburgers. We usually got five for a dollar, which made one for each of us and one extra for the driver. An occasional indulgence was a can of weak beer. It was gradually dawning on us that a few hundred dollars would not go far even at that rate.

Inexpensive breakfast was eaten by the roadside, and comprised delicious fruit such as strawberries, with cereal and "half and half", that is half full-cream milk and half skim milk, eaten from paper plates with plastic spoons. At a drugstore lunch stop by the side of the highway in Flagstaff, Arizona, we encountered the American side salad.

Unlike the Australian chopped lettuce delicacy of the day, it was a routine course accompanying the simplest meal. On taking one's order, the waitress always said: "ItalianFrenchRoquefortorThousandIslands"? It took us quite a while to work out this language and to give a coherent reply. As we had a simple lunch the mighty freight trains rolled by, a mile or two in length, much longer than we had ever seen before.

On across the great arid lands of the south-western United States we drove, enjoying, albeit briefly, the Zion and Bryce National Parks, the Grand Canyon, the Petrified Forest, and the Painted Desert National Parks. We experienced a little bit of the Spanish past of Santa Fe and some historic buildings in Albuquerque before driving down through the eroded Badlands of the Texas Panhandle. Dallas greeted us with its gleaming towers in the bright clear light. Eventually, weary from a long trip, we drove into Houston and checked in to a fancy motel. We soon escaped when we recognised what the tariff was. When I reported at work, there were a few listings of lodgings which had been used by other staff members in the past and we managed to find a cheap apartment on the wrong side of town.

Houston

The Americans have a talent for building inexpensive accommodation. This place did prove adequate for our needs, but we were always a bit suspicious of the .45 calibre hole in the bed head and a brown stain on the mattress. Next day I had to front up at Methodist Hospital for my baptism of fire with the great man, Michael DeBakey.

Michael DeBakey

I had met Mike DeBakey several years earlier, when hc visited Sydney and delivered a lecture at the BMA building in Macquarie Street. He was a remarkably fluent speaker and illustrated his work with the most brilliant photographs, movies and charts, which were to become a hallmark of the Baylor University Medical School. I learned later that it was Mike's sister Lois, a medical librarian, who edited every document that came out of that institution to stamp it with the corporate style.

That evening back in Sydney, DeBakey presented his results, and the audience members were gobsmacked by the sheer volume of work that he had done and the excellence of the results in such a very high risk field. I was sitting behind Alan Sharp, then Senior Vascular Surgeon at Sydney Hospital, and heard him scoff: "Nobody can possibly have done that many operations".

Now here I was on my first morning in Houston, keen to make a good impression. I was quickly grabbed by Arthur Beall, a junior staff member at

Baylor, whom I had met earlier in Sydney. He said: "Quick! Change into your greens, he'll be here in a minute".

The Operating Schedule was written on a giant blackboard occupying a whole wall of the lobby of the operating room suite. I ran my eye down the list and thought it a solid week's work. I soon found out it was in fact for that one day and, like every day, it contained two or three or more open heart operations, three or four abdominal aneurysms, and a handful of operations for obstructive arterial disease; usually about fifteen in all. Each one of those is a very big operation and most surgeons would need half a day for each. Mike had several operating rooms, and plenty of assistants, as well as a couple of excellent junior associates. That made for efficient use of his time as he could run from room to room, doing key parts of most operations himself. It was clear how Mike had accumulated those incredible numbers of cases.

I soon got to meet DeBakey's associates and to learn their strong points. Ed Garrett was an unflappable man, calm amidst the storm, apparently immune to fatigue, and a friendly supporter of the trainees. I quickly made a deal with Ed to the effect that whenever any patient needed a reoperation, which usually occurred at night, he could call me in to be his assistant. This was a stroke of genius, as it is the cases that go wrong from which one learns nearly everything important.

Jimmy Howell was a tall skinny boy from the backwoods of Louisiana. He loved to play the country hick, but in fact was a very intelligent surgeon. This was his first job after completion of training; he was a hard worker and a good one. He remained on the staff for the rest of his career and became probably the best coronary surgeon of them all.

Mike DeBakey was surely the most famous surgeon of the 20th Century, and he fully lived up to his reputation as what my friend Giancarlo Rastelli used classify as a tenore, or tenor, that is a shouter.

DeBakey was born to a Lebanese immigrant family in Louisiana, and attended Tulane Medical School in New Orleans. As a medical student he invented the roller pump which became one of the key components of the heart-lung machine which later made open heart surgery possible. Among his achievements with the US Surgeon General's office in WW2 was the idea of forward surgical teams, which evolved into the MASH concept in Korea. He invented or refined many of the basic techniques of arterial surgery and developed many of the instruments and materials which made it possible. His associate, Ed Garrett, used say: “If it ain't called DeBakey it ain't got a name”.

DeBakey was ugly, short and stooped, but physically powerful and tireless. He had the unusual ability not to need much sleep, and, as he wasted no time on leisure, he was able to do two full days' work in 24 hours. Sometimes the long day's operating started calmly but it was seldom long before something or someone precipitated a fit of abusive shouting, recriminations, and, on a bad day, a sacking. His sallow face, pale from lack of sunlight, became suffused to match his mood and demeanour, hence his nickname of Black Mike. When he shouted “You're fired!” there was no redress, as the Prof was the Chief, and all powerful. I mused, if that is the word when someone is yelling abuse two feet from you, on Lord Acton's dictum that “all power corrupts”. Why, I wondered, would so talented and exalted a teacher stoop to such crass bullying.

Mike was very intelligent, a brilliant organiser, publicist and promoter, politically well-connected in Texas and Washington, energetic and adept and a creative innovator. Like most of my colleagues I had to be prepared to take what came as I had relocated with my family halfway around the world to learn all I could at the centre of my growing specialty.

Stanley Crawford

After six months of unremitting toil under the supervision of DeBakey, the next three months term with Stanley Crawford was a pleasure. Stan had a reputation as an all-round good man, a reg'lar guy as they used to say, a very hard worker but fair, generous, and amusing. Another piece of good fortune was to share this term with an East German friend, Peter Thiele. Peter and his mother had somehow escaped to West Germany, where he attended Medical School at Heidelberg. On receiving his Fellowship to Houston, he taught himself English from a Berlitz tape within a couple of weeks. His speech was sometimes amusingly accented but served him well. We liked him very much, and he became a frequent visitor at our house for dinner. Stan enjoyed taunting us that, as an Australian and a German, all we were good for was beer drinking. It is true that after Peter found a source of Lowenbrau, we did seal our friendship with an occasional can of that excellent beverage.

Stanley Crawford was another Southerner who liked to affect a rustic image. He was, indeed, a country boy but as a distinguished graduate of Harvard Medical School he was no backwoodsman. His hillbilly mannerisms and Southern speech patterns endeared him to the local patients. He loved to hunt. Whenever we came upon a patient who was a farmer from the neighbouring areas of East Texas or Louisiana, it would not take long before the boss made some innocent query along the lines of: "Saaay, I bet you-all have got some fine dogs out on that farm of yours". Almost invariably, the farmer would soon be bragging about his bird-dogs, and extending an invitation to Stan to bring his gun so that he could assess the dogs' talents.

One weekend we knew that Stanley was going with some friends to hunt birds in Mexico. Next Monday we were quick to ask if he had any luck. He announced, "We shot 200 doves and three Mexicans". His explanation was that the Mexicans had been sitting in an irrigation ditch and sprang up at the wrong time, receiving a few stray pellets.

Because he was third on the seniority totem pole at the Methodist Hospital, when he was setting up practice Stanley had needed to give extraordinarily good service to his referring doctors, and he in his turn continued to repay their loyalty even after he had become world-famous and extremely busy. So every couple of weeks we got the opportunity to go with him to one of the smaller cities in Texas to do one or more operations. We had to show up in front of his house at six o'clock in the morning to join him in his white Thunderbird, of which he was very proud, and head off across the countryside at breakneck speed. We would stop somewhere along the way for a quick breakfast.

Operating in a strange environment is always challenging, but Stan was very good at improvising with whatever instruments and materials were to hand. The patients and their doctors got superb service, which would otherwise have been unaffordable for them.

Another of Stanley's old supporters was a local osteopathic surgeon; yes, there were such animals in Texas at that time. Sadly, over the years, this man's alcoholism had got the best of him, so he had no choice but to call on a loyal supporter such as Stan to do his major operations. In the circumstances, Stanley greatly appreciated the opportunity to bring a burly German and substantial Australian to provide a buffer between the patient, Stanley, and the sozzled supporter.

One thing that all surgical assistants agree upon is their hatred of the Deaver's retractor. This is a large, spatula-like instrument that is used to hold organs out of the way to allow access to the operative field. Its handle is a flat, blade-like metal strip. If you hold it at all firmly, it is soon very uncomfortable and after a little longer, the fingers go numb because of pressure. As we often used to say: "Deaver never did any assisting". Our favourite scrub nurse, called Sally, was married to a dentistry student. We prevailed on him to drill a hole in the bottom of a glass beer mug which we screwed onto a strip of metal about the same size and shape as a Deaver. Sally packed it up and sterilised it just like any instrument. On the last day that we operated with Stan Crawford, as soon as he called for this instrument, she handed him our beer mug retractor. He laughed uproariously, and chuckled for the rest of the day. I hope that was a good parting memory for him of his devoted German and Aussie admirers.

Denton Cooley

Everyone wanted to work for Denton Cooley. He graduated from the University of Texas before studying Medicine at Johns Hopkins Medical School. He had been a basketball player, tall, blonde and handsome, and still excelled at golf and tennis, although he rarely had time to play them.

Shortly before my time he had fallen out with Michael DeBakey, no doubt because he baulked at the restrictions imposed on him by the Old Man. In truth, no town was big enough for the two of them. Thus he had set up his own surgical programme across the parking lot, at St Luke's and Texas Children's Hospital. In retaliation, Mike restricted his access to the pool of trainees and residents, so Peter Thiele and I were in for a mighty busy three months. This was especially so as summer was coming on and this was a convenient time for children to have their operations. The workload was enormous.

Despite the hectic pace we got through all our work with good humour. The boss was almost always relaxed, and frequently given to cracking jokes. There were a few funny cartoons around the operating room, one which showed a spectacularly simian Michael DeBakey saying to his Resident: "I like your idea, son, I am glad I thought of it".

A portable radio played music from one of the numerous local FM stations. The cheery rhythms of Al Hirt's trumpet were ideal to maintain an up-tempo while we closed the incisions. There would be just time for a quick cup of bitter coffee before running in to scrub for the next case.

Cooley was famed for his speed, which he achieved without appearing to move quickly, or, indeed, hardly moving at all. The secret, which is easier said than done, is to be so systematic as to waste no movements. "Do it once, do it right" or "Do it right—the first time!"

These were the principles which I strove to perfect in later years, to analyse each operation, cut out all unnecessary steps, and standardise the performance so there was no need to rush.

Denton had many funny sayings, most of which do not bear repeating. Often a visitor would ask him: "Dr Cooley, how do you account for being so fast?" He would reply: "I figure, when they go on the pump they start to die and I've gotta beat them to it."

Cooley also exemplified the entrepreneurial spirit of the best Americans. After my time, as his practice grew to enormous volume, he built the Texas Heart Institute on the campus of St Luke's, essentially a large private hospital devoted to his personal practice.

As a side line he put his capital into a new Bank which he modestly named the Bank of Texas. Later he built a large hotel adjacent to the hospital for visitors and relatives. This venture got into financial trouble during the "oil shock" recession of the '70s and he was for a time in Chapter 11 bankruptcy. That does not carry the same stigma as in Australia, and in no time he had solved the difficulties and gone on to greater strengths.

Mayo Clinic

The final crazy quarter of my year in Houston finally came to an end and it was time to drive north to Minnesota and the famed Mayo Clinic. We packed a U-Haul trailer with our meagre possessions, piled into the old two-tone green Mercury once more, and headed towards Oklahoma. Forty-five miles per hour was our limit with a trailer, and it was about all I cared to try. By Kansas I had taken off my ten-gallon hat and put it on the seat; by Iowa it was underneath the seat.

Onward through the wheat and cornfields, where we caught our first sight of the giant silos towering above the small townships. Further along were the great red hip-roofed barns characteristic of the Midwest.

It was a scramble to get organised and for me to get to work on the Monday morning. I found I was in fact overdue, and did not escape from the hospital for a couple of days. It fell to Marilyn to select an apartment in a nice area towards the edge of town and not far from Silver Lake. This was an artificial lake, made by damming the Zumbro River to provide cooling for the local power station. Hence it never completely froze over in winter and therefore provided a sanctuary for the Greater Canada geese which wintered there.

Our apartment was nearly new and, most importantly, had central heating which was taken care of by somebody else. This was a significant consideration in this climate.

Climate is one of many striking differences between Northern and Southern conditions and cultures. In the fierce Minnesota winter the temperature can drop to minus 40 Fahrenheit (coincidentally minus 40C). Spring, following the thaw in May, is very beautiful as trees come out in bud, and birds and flowers reappear. They say you can play golf in summer, if it falls on 4 July! Before too long the crops are ripening, long skeins of great Canada geese appear honking in the sky, and snow is not far away. Quite a change from the steamy heat of the Gulf Coast of Texas.

Climate is not the only difference. There are great historical, cultural, and language distinctions between the South and Southwest and that of the Midwest of the United States. In general, Southerners do not accept that they lost the Civil War. Even the children know that "Goddam Yankee" is really one word. While the Northern speakers roll that r-r-r sound, the true Southerners hardly pronounce it at all. Southerners cuss a lot but Northerners rarely swear and often take their religion seriously. The Midwest has a strong Protestant feel to it, derived from the largely Scandinavian and German Lutheran settlers. They used to say in Rochester that on Sundays even the Unitarians put on their best suits and then don't go to church.

I should write a few words about the Mayo Clinic, "The Clinic in the Cornfields". Outside of medical circles most people who know of it have heard a big fib, as they associate the name with various crazy diets which have nothing to do with the Clinic and are a nagging embarrassment to it. This extraordinary institution grew from a general practice in the small midwestern town of Rochester, Minnesota about the end of the 19th Century.

In due course old Doctor Mayo was joined by his sons, Will and Charlie, in an early form of group practice. Their reputation was built on high-quality, low mortality surgery for such common endemic problems as thyrotoxic goitre. They quickly attracted other doctors to the practice, were early advocates of specialisation, and recruited radiologists and leaders in other specialties as they developed. Excellent results and efficient service made for a profitable practice and there was no income tax in those days, so the business side expanded and prospered.

By 1914 they had built their first clinic building, a three-floor redbrick cube that is still in use. Another important contributing event was a severe tornado, which devastated the town and took many lives. From this tragedy arose St Mary's Hospital, still one of the major institutions associated with the Clinic.

Doctor Will, as he was called, was not only a safe surgeon but also a genius of organisation and administration. Before long he enticed the Methodist Church to build their hospital a mile away from St Mary's, engendering plenty of genteel competition. In due course, hotels grew up around the clinic to service the needs of the visitors, and also numerous guesthouses for the less affluent visitors. Such is the level of organisation that the footpaths around the Clinic are warmed by steam to rid them of snow in winter, and the Clinic is linked to the major hotels by tunnels.

There was already a railroad running through the town and it became the fashion for the well-to-do to travel long distances for their annual check-up or treatments. An international airport was later developed, capable of handling jet aircraft.

The clinic continues to grow and to do excellent work. One of the favourite questions asked of the staff at the clinic is: "How many doctors actually work at the Mayo Clinic?" My friend the Paediatric Cardiologist Don Ritter used to chuckle as he would reply: "Oh, about 50 per cent of them!"

This great institution dominates the small city out in the flat farmlands of Minnesota, its buildings towering over the traditional white weatherboard houses with their two compact storeys and a storm cellar.

By the time we were living there, the IBM Corporation had established a large research Institute outside the town. The Clinic, the hospitals and IBM dominate the community, attracting many doctors and engineers, and employing lots of the hardworking locals. Rochester was a wealthy community with about 50,000 inhabitants, with excellent municipal facilities, schools, community theatre and the like.

Reflecting the laws of supply and demand, Mayo paid very frugal stipends to its trainees. I was very fortunate to be awarded an Overseas Fellowship by the National Heart Foundation of Australia. This included a reasonable living allowance so we were no longer completely living on the breadline.

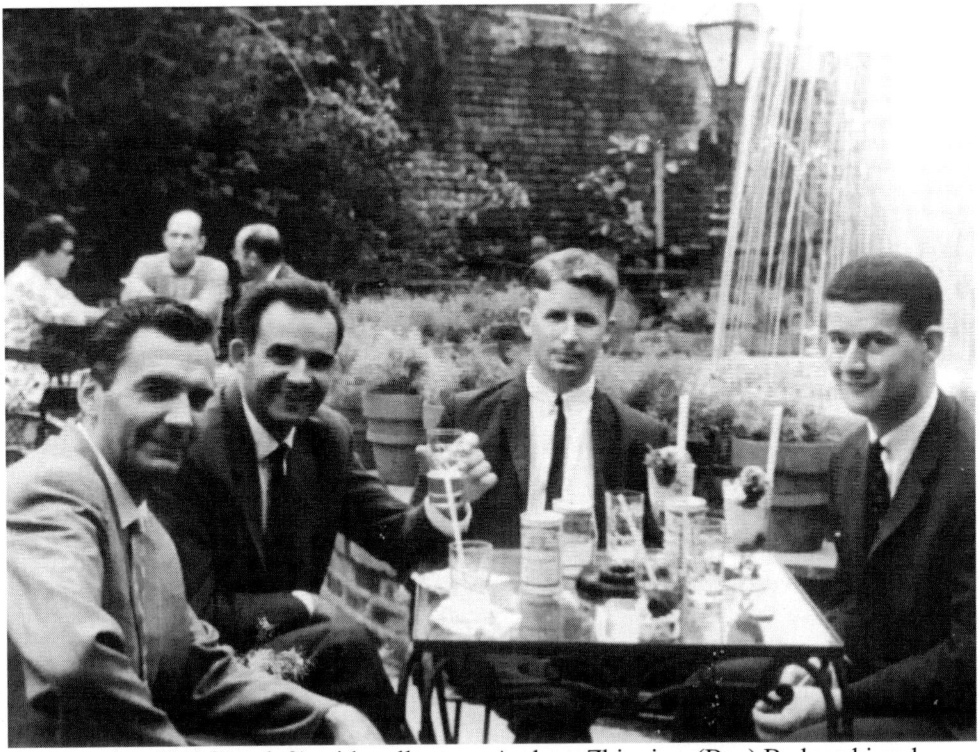

Tim third from left) with colleagues Andree, Zbigniew (Ben) Bednarski and Peter Thiele at Pat O'Brien's Bar in New Orleans in 1964

John Kirklin

I went to the Mayo Clinic to study with John Kirklin. He began training as a Neurosurgeon but saw the potential of Cardiac Surgery. He spent several years in painstaking preliminary scientific work and, in collaboration with IBM, developed a sophisticated and highly automated heart-lung machine.

As sometimes happens in Medicine, the whole field was given a kick forward with Walt Lillehei at the University of Minnesota in Minneapolis. Walt went ahead and jumped the gun, performing the first open heart operations with cross-circulation, using a parent to act as heart-lung machine for their child. This caused plenty of medical tut-tutting; it was said to have been the first operation in history with a potential mortality rate of 200 per cent!

Kirklin quickly followed with his machine, and before long had overtaken everyone both in number of operations and the excellence of his results. He was just the person for the job, painstaking, obsessive, industrious and uncompromising. When I worked with him, he was about 48 years old, slightly built, with an iron-grey crew cut, dapper in dress and manner. This precision extended to his manners of speech and writing which were deliberate and meticulous. He was fond of adverbs, and I for one agreed that a liberal use of words such as "precisely" and "accurately" could bring even scientific writing alive.

Nowadays he would be called a control freak, and people either loved him or hated him. I was in the former camp and came to admire him very much. He was a careful and methodical operator, a great systematic thinker and organiser but not overly original. Whenever new ideas appeared he would evaluate them in a diligent scientific way, whether by experiment, by close observation of our own results, or by basic research informed by detailed consultation with the relevant specialists. John Kirklin literally wrote the book on cardiac surgery, in two large tomes co-authored with Sir Brian Barratt-Boyes of Auckland. They analysed and presented their combined huge experience in a way that can never again be reproduced.

My cigar-smoking friend, George Daicoff from Chicago used say of him "Koiklin is an example of the American woik ethic gone crazy!" He even pursued his recreational equestrian sport of dressage obsessively, riding his horse by night after a long day's work. We joked that in the long, dark, subzero winter when all the other animals were reclining in a warm barn, Kirklin's horse would have to go through its paces again and again, precisely and accurately, until the performance was "just right".

Surgery at the Mayo Clinic was systematic and highly organised. Each surgical team would operate on alternate days, and on the non-surgery day would conduct formal rounds, check on post-operative patients in the clinic, see consultations, and attend to correspondence and other administrative details. The Fellows (equivalent to interns and residents) would begin the day at half past six in the morning with a detailed round of all their hospital inpatients, checking all results and ensuring that the records were in perfect shape. We would then meet the boss for breakfast in the staff dining room at half past seven and follow that by rounds at eight o'clock. Every detail would be checked and commented upon and corrected where necessary. Kirklin would then conduct an informal seminar, testing our knowledge, inculcating any new ideas and generally enlightening us on the latest thinking in his specialty. The First Assistant would then accompany him to the Clinic building downtown and participate in consultations with the physicians, where decisions would be made and surgery arranged.

Operating days were long but efficient. The team would meet in the surgical suite, and the boss would sit down and review the medical record of each patient for the day, detailing any particular requirements for anaesthesia, monitoring or care. The first major case would get underway and the team for the second operating room would sneak off for a cup of coffee before being called to start the second case when the first one was "off bypass", that is when the main part of the operation was completed.

Dr Kirklin and most of his colleagues preferred to do four operations between the two rooms, which would take up most of a long day but be manageable. At the end of each operation the assistants would accompany the patient to the cardiac intensive care area, settle them in, and begin the intensive observations which were the key to safe post-operative management. If everything was satisfactory, we could sometimes get some sleep in a room that had been assigned to us.

I spent two years with Dr Kirklin. For the first quarter my grand title was that of Second Assistant, a general dogsbody, fetcher and carrier, performer of menial duties, and, yes, Second Assistant at operations. No different, really, from what an intern does anywhere else, but a humbling experience for someone who had done it all eight years before and been qualified as a surgeon for several years. The time was soon over and it was my turn to be First Assistant for six months. In this great job one really does assist the great man at every operation, as well as steadying the ship and supervising the Second Assistant, watching the patients like a hawk and generally being the eyes and ears of the boss when he is out of sight.

At my request Dr Kirklin arranged for me to spend three months in the cardiac catheterisation laboratory at St Mary's Hospital, another stroke of good luck. The head of the lab was Jeremy Swan, a peppery Irishman who, although he was about to move to the West Coast, still exerted his personality over the performance and standards of his department. Day-to-day management fell to Shabhudin Rahimtoola, Sabu for short, a bright Pakistani doctor with the highest standards. My fellow learners were budding medical cardiologists, and I had an advantage over them in that I had many surgical skills which they lacked and which occasionally came in handy. Most of all, I learned how cardiologists think and how these diagnostic procedures are done, how they can be interpreted and hence how reliable they are. That advantage stayed with me for the next 40 years.

In my second year my title was Research Assistant to Doctor Kirklin. I participated in two major studies, one of which was to report the results of all the ventricular septal defect operations he had performed to that point, making me for a while the world authority on the subject. I analysed the records of over 400 patients who had been operated upon, followed them up in detail, had them return for re-evaluation and if necessary cardiac catheterisation, and published the results.

This sometimes mundane task was a window into the development of the thinking of world-leading cardiologists, physiologists, pathologists, and surgeons. Part of the task was to review the world literature to that time. Here the superb organisation of the medical library came into play.

It is interesting to reflect on how important this library was, before any automated or Google-like technology was available. The collection of books and journals occupied two full floors of the historic Plummer building, which had been built in the 1930s as the first high-rise Clinic tower. To maximise the efficiency of literature searching, the Clinic provided expert librarians who would locate the necessary publications and place them in an allotted carrel to be perused whenever time was available. To sit at the window high above the city and immerse oneself in study, undistracted by other tasks, was sheer luxury. To do it while snow drifted down outside was a rare pleasure.

I presented the completed work at a meeting of the American Association for Thoracic Surgery in Vancouver, and it was generously received. The slides illustrating my talk had been prepared by the Department of Publications, also a major service within the Plummer building. We could call on the services of photographers, medical illustrators, and people to prepare the slides to the exacting standards required by the Clinic. Kirklin and I rewrote my draft manuscript several times, and the final paper was published in the *Journal of Thoracic Surgery* (now called *The Journal of Cardiothoracic Surgery*).

IBM

My second job was to collaborate with IBM engineer Louis Sheppard on the use of computers in the post-operative care of patients. Sheppard was an excellent colleague and taught me a lot about the computers of those days. Our pride and joy was an IBM System 360, shared by the whole Clinic, occupying an entire floor of the Harwick building which housed all the medical records of the Mayo Clinic. Our then state-of-the-art computer had much less computing power than a modern mobile phone, and we communicated with it using decks of punch-cards. Sheppard programmed the computer in its Fortran language, although that language was really intended for mathematical purposes.

By the mid-1960s, computers were beginning to be used in industry for automatic process control, especially in boring, repetitive, dirty or dangerous tasks requiring infallible precision, such as in chemical factories or mines. Patient monitoring promised to be one such task. But beyond acquiring, storing and presenting data, our project aimed to "close the loop" by automating the patient treatment including infusion of drugs to improve cardiac function. In this way Lou Shepherd and I defined many of the possible ways in which computers could be used to improve the safety and reliability of patient care. Dr Kirklin subsequently incorporated these ideas in his new Department at University of Alabama in Mobile, Alabama.

An interesting minor project was the automation of blood pressure measurement using a pneumatic cuff; that is to automate the familiar Korotkoff BP measurement process. Chances are your doctor records your BP using such a system today, and it no longer costs several million dollars; you can buy it at the pharmacy for a few bucks.

When I look back on my time with Kirklin I admire his numerous talents and value the things I learned. He was a master of sustained, controlled, disciplined work, with a great talent for concentrating on a single task at a time. And, somewhat surprisingly, another important thing I discovered was that I would not choose to be exactly like him even if I had the talent and the opportunity.

Chapter 5: Return to Australia

Three years in America were drawing to a close and I needed to plan my future. Remaining in the United States might have been attractive but I did not seriously consider it. I had a strong sense of attachment and obligation to Australia, especially considering the extent to which all my education beyond primary school had been supported by bursaries, scholarships, research grants and fellowships.

The major awards were:

- NSW State Bursary supported tuition and board at Hurlstone Agricultural High School
- NSW State Bursary supported tuition at Sydney University Medical School, board at St Andrew's College, a book allowance and a small living allowance
- In 1950 the Bursary was superseded by a new Commonwealth Scholarship Scheme, introduced by the Menzies Government and available to all who matriculated to university
- NSW Cancer Council Research Grant supported my project from 1961 to 1963
- Fulbright Scholarship, a US Government scheme, funded travel to the US
- Australian Heart Foundation Travelling Fellowship provided living expenses for two years in the US.

Royal Prince Alfred Hospital

General Superintendent Edgar Thompson and his Assistant Don Child invited me back to Royal Prince Alfred Hospital as a salaried Staff Specialist. This was welcome, but I was not reassured of the necessary support. I had considered a post in Singapore and also a position which had become available in Brisbane, where the Chermside unit had been struggling with indifferent results. Within a couple of months, the Singapore job was taken by one of their Chinese candidates while the Brisbane post was accepted by Mark O'Brien, a well-trained Melbourne surgeon who proved to be an excellent choice. With some trepidation, I signed up with Prince Alfred.

Nearly all heart surgeons worldwide were employed full-time with some professional salary support. In their different ways, professional arrangements in the UK, Scandinavia, Europe, USA and Canada all provided either academic or salaried systems. The Green Lane Hospital Cardiac Unit in Auckland, which had been established by Douglas Robb and developed by Rowan Nicks and then Brian Barratt-Boyes, was a small-country version of what I considered an ideal working arrangement. Talented salaried full-time specialists in various disciplines including Surgery, Cardiology, Radiology, Anaesthesia, Medical Technologies and some basic sciences worked in a cooperative and mutually supportive milieu and were doing excellent work.

That model could never have succeeded at Prince Alfred. The Administration at that time lacked interest in strategic development and did not understand that infrastructure and support are essential for major projects [In subsequent years they developed many excellent facilities]. There were also problems with conflicting personalities in the Cardiothoracic Surgery department.

Soon after open heart surgery got underway in 1957, Frank Mills withdrew due to health problems to concentrate on General Surgery and Paul Tomlinson retired. Sandy Grant was a good Thoracic Surgeon who became a proficient Cardiac Surgeon with little interest in or enthusiasm for academic matters. Rowan Nicks supported me generously but was often perceived as an impractical dreamer. Bruce Leckie had recently returned from the UK and was a successful, entrepreneurial Thoracic Surgeon with no pretence at scholarship.

After an uneasy period of unemployment, I accepted the job of Staff Specialist in Cardiac Surgery at Prince Alfred. There was considerable goodwill from many people but little practical support or infrastructure. With some difficulty I found a small room in the Page Chest Pavilion to use as an office but had no clerical or technical staff.

The fundamental problem was that there was not sufficient work for the number of heart surgeons at Prince Alfred. Too many people were chasing too few operations. Rowan Nicks, in one of his typically generous gestures, assigned all of his cardiac operative patients to me and he assisted me with their procedures.

We still had no house in Sydney, so Marilyn and the children were living with her parents in Gosford. Don Child generously offered me use of a VIP visitor's room in the old Residents' Quarters and I lived there for some months, visiting the family at weekends, until we bought a house in Eastwood early the following year. I enjoyed the social contact with the hospital's Resident staff but all in all it was an unhappy period.

Royal Alexandra Hospital for Children

Douglas Cohen was my salvation. One morning in early 1967 I was surprised by a phone call from anaesthetist Dr Graham Fisk, who asked me to meet him in the operating theatre at the Royal Alexandra Hospital for Children (RAHC, often shortened to The Children's Hospital, or Kids). Dr Douglas Cohen was in the midst of an operation and having difficulty in interpreting his findings. Fisk met me at the fire stairs, showed me to the change room, and introduced me to the team in Operating Room 4.

I quickly reviewed the medical record and all the available data and examined the heart as it lay exposed within the chest. The preoperative diagnosis was inaccurate, so I could not contribute much to the problem at hand. A couple of months later, however, Dr Cohen asked me in for a little chat.

Douglas Cohen

Douglas Cohen was a middle-aged, affable, established paediatric surgeon with an academic bent. He had successfully established the open-heart surgery program at the Children's Hospital in 1959. Early results were good, but by 1967 there was some difficulty in reaching the next level of complexity. It was arranged that I should be seconded to do one operation list per week there, later increasing to two per week. In 1969, when Cohen unfortunately suffered a serious myocardial infarction, I took over as Head of Cardiac Surgery at RAHC. I maintained my contact with Prince Alfred and continued to operate one list a week there for many more years. With the retirement of Rowan Nicks, the return of Doug Baird after completing his overseas training, and my eventual appointment to the newly opened Westmead (adult) Teaching Hospital, I relinquished all further duties at Prince Alfred.

One of Cohen's many talents was his ability to assemble a capable team and to attract community support for this new and expensive endeavour. Sir Adolf Basser, a successful Sydney jeweller and philanthropist, funded the Adolf Basser Institute of Cardiology and purchased much of the early equipment. Cohen's sailing friend and engineer, Vivian Ebsary, had built a surface cooling apparatus for surgery under hypothermia. Cohen used this for coarctation repair and also for repair of atrial septal defect under inflow occlusion.

[Coarctation is a severe congenital narrowing of the aorta beyond the origin of the branches to the head, neck and upper limbs, causing high blood pressure in the upper body. The operation requires temporary clamping above and below the narrowed segment to allow removal of the narrow portion and resuturing of the normal aorta. Atrial septal defect occurs when a normal opening between the right and left atria, or collecting chambers, fails to close after birth. Inflow occlusion allowed the heart to empty, permitting a few minutes in which to repair such simple defects. Refer to fuller descriptions elsewhere in this memoir.]

Ebsary built, at his Brookvale works, a very high quality heart-lung machine. This was a solid chassis containing a strong electric motor to drive the hydraulic system providing power to the DeBakey pumps and an oxygenator. The oxygenator was based on the Kay-Cross rotating disc model. Blood flowed through the lower third of a horizontal Pyrex cylinder in which a series of steel discs, each about the size of a CD, rotated through the pool of blood to lift a capillary film and expose it to an O2/CO2 atmosphere. Oxygenators came in a range of sizes from 8 inches long for small children up to 36 inches long for an adult. The discs were hand polished stainless steel of the highest quality and finish and the ancillary components were similarly professionally built. In time, the disc oxygenator was superseded by a bubble oxygenator, but we continued to use that pump chassis for many years.

Adolph Basser Institute of Cardiology

After the frustrations of my early experiences at Royal Prince Alfred, the set up and staff of the Adolph Basser Institute of Cardiology at the Children's Hospital were a relief. It was just as I had been accustomed to seeing at the Mayo Clinic, though on a much smaller scale. Our facilities were adequate and a talented multidisciplinary team worked happily and effectively together.

Our senior Honorary Physician, Douglas Stuckey, was a cardiologist of the old school; a sound clinician and competent at cardiac catheterisation. He was a reliable and loyal colleague at all times.

John Celermajer was simply a genius, a man of high energy, high intelligence, and highly concentrated activity. John's boyhood was spent in hiding with his Jewish family in Lvov, then in Poland [now Lviv, Ukraine]. John's sister did not survive the German occupation. He sometimes enjoyed telling the story of how, at the end of the war, his father stole a truck to drive the family to a new life in France. John had his formal schooling in Paris, in a new language of French. When he was 16 the family migrated to Australia and settled in Sydney. John completed his secondary schooling at Sydney Boys High School, in yet another new language of English, graduating dux of the school and top student in every subject except English.

At Sydney University Medical School John excelled and graduated with the University's Gold Medal.

As a Junior Resident at Royal Prince Alfred Hospital he bore this outstanding academic reputation without much humility. Transferring to the Children's Hospital at Camperdown, he thrived as Resident Medical Officer, Registrar, and Chief Resident Medical Officer, excelling in all the paediatric subspecialties but eventually settling on Paediatric Cardiology as his special interest.

When I joined the Children's Hospital in 1967, Celermajer was absent, pursuing a Fellowship under the tutelage of Richard Rowe at the Johns Hopkins Hospital in Baltimore. After this "finishing school" experience he returned to Sydney and re-joined the Adolph Basser Institute of Cardiology, soon being promoted to Director. With his old friend Denby Bowdler, the Director of Radiology, John and I formed an excellent team of complementary specialists, soon to be joined by anaesthetist John Overton.

Celermajer was a near perfect consultant physician with whom to work. Having evaluated a patient he would have arrived at a clear and precisely expressed diagnosis which almost always was accurate or very close. He would state his provisional diagnosis and enunciate a proposed course of action. Where more specialised tests or procedures were required, he would set them out precisely. By that time there were many conditions for which we had established fairly standardised management principles. In the occasional event that we did not agree on the proposed course of action we would decide what was necessary to resolve the uncertainty — usually some further test or piece of information.

Post operatively, we always debriefed frankly and in detail on each case, confirming those things that had proven correct and learning what needed to be learned from any that were not. John was an excellent colleague during post-operative management. He was diligent in following his cases and forthcoming in any further suggestions about the management. Win or lose, I never knew him to second-guess his opinions or otherwise act as a "Monday morning quarterback".

Whether at work or socially, he never seemed really relaxed. Almost every discussion was treated as a debate. I assumed that this was a legacy of his French education and reflected the French love of Cartesian dialectic. Maybe it is a Jewish attribute as well. Either way, he could not resist an intellectual contest, loved to win, and bore no ill will on the rare occasions that he lost.

John's overwhelming personal attributes were high intelligence, high energy, obsessive punctilio and unfailing attention to detail. His time management was extraordinary, allowing him to live a fulfilling personal life beyond work. As well as the long hours and great effort which he devoted to his job, he spent almost as much effort and energy on leisure and family.

He and Tina had two children. David, who is now an extraordinary cardiologist and researcher, had the fortune to inherit his father's intelligence and his mother's charm. Daniela, whom I do not know well, is an academic in the life sciences.

John enjoyed the performing arts and many fine arts, especially antiques and paintings. His collection of Australian paintings graced his house. He still had time for golf and simply adored his motorcars, even the Jaguar which so often failed to start.

His leukaemia diagnosis came as a dreadful shock, but he fought it with his usual stubbornness and rarely permitted the symptoms or the treatment to disrupt his energetic life. Years went by and it sometimes seemed that he could beat the odds. As so often, the final acute phase of the illness was swift and distressing. True to character he continued to work right to the last few days of his life, saying that if he was going to be miserable, he preferred to be miserable doing something he enjoyed.

John's legacy includes the thousands of patients for whom he cared. He was an outstanding teacher, with special talent in passing on his skills of clinical diagnosis. His stewardship of the Adolf Basser Institute of Cardiology was sound and his teamwork contributed a great deal to the effectiveness of our multidisciplinary approach.

It was a privilege to have worked so long and so closely with John Celermajer. He was a marvellous doctor and a man of contrasts. He was vain, selfish and egocentric in some ways yet remarkably generous in others. So clever and inventive himself, he thought politics could be influenced by logic. He had a tin ear, but came to love Mozart.

Another colleague, Don Gengos, Staff Specialist Cardiac Surgeon, had grown up in Moree. Having chosen Paediatric Surgery, he was swept up in the early years of the cardiac subspecialty. He was clever at management and had instituted many of the systems at the Adolph Basser Institute of Cardiology. Don was garrulous, affable, and sociable. After some years he decided not to persist with clinical surgery and instead became a "Medical Director" for a drug company. Business life suited him, and later he moved permanently to the US to be International Medical Director of Eli Lilly Corporation and abandoned clinical medicine altogether.

Denby Bowdler had trained in radiology at the Children's Hospital and was thrust into the position of Director of Radiology when the incumbent, Dr Paddy Grattan-Smith, resigned. Driven, perhaps overly conscientious, Denby was a very competent diagnostic radiologist and fitted well with the rest of the team.

Graham Fisk was well versed in Paediatric Anaesthesia, having trained at Alder Hay Children's Hospital in Liverpool, UK. He managed the anaesthesia and cardiopulmonary bypass with care and precision. His rigid views on medicine and life could sometimes be irritating but one could always count on his skill and devotion.

Philomena Clifton was a quintessentially obsessive, highly conscientious old-style Nursing Sister. She had cared for Cohen's cardiac patients from the beginning, and was in charge of the Peter McDonald Cardiac Surgery

Intensive Therapy Unit when I joined. No errors were tolerated and everything had to be perfect, even down to the technique of folding the children's garments. This trait can be irritating and frustrating at times, but when the chips are down it is helpful to know that someone is utterly reliable. Maybe she sometimes let perfect be the enemy of good, as the saying goes. After several years I discovered that she was still working into the night to summarise the fluid balance charts, long after the anaesthetist who had originally requested this work had left the staff. No matter; she was loyal and utterly devoted to the welfare of the children.

John Jackson was an unusual and valuable team member. He had suffered from tuberculous disease of the spine as a child, spending years as an inpatient in the Children's Hospital. He had become something of a favourite with the administration, who recognised his technical knack and gave him a job as the electrocardiograph technician just before he turned 16. As well as his facility with electronics, he was a self-taught fitter and turner and general fixer of things and became our chief technician. Somewhere along the way he 'got religion", carrying his Testament with him at all times and generally exerting a gentle steadying influence on the team. In the early days he not only maintained our electronic equipment, but built a lot of it himself. When new perfusion equipment was installed, it often required customisation, and John would turn up brass fittings on the lathe so we always had a most professional looking and functioning apparatus.

Another key early staff member was Paul Bernhardt, a self-taught young English technical officer. He had a flair for electronics, and later computers, and learned many tricks of the trade from his boss, John Jackson.

Of the Staff Anaesthetists already on the team when I joined, Graham Fisk, whom I mentioned above, transferred after a couple of years to the Prince of Wales Children's Hospital. Fortunately, we had by then been joined by John Overton. Verlie Lines remained a stalwart supporter until her untimely death some 20 years later.

Three Visiting Anaesthetists who were already involved were Serge Bodlander, Richard Bailey, and Jeanette Thirlwell. Bodlander withdrew after a short time and confined his efforts mostly to Royal Prince Alfred. Bailey and Thirlwell continued to give their excellent technical and moral support until my retirement at the end of 1997 – 30 years of friendly collaboration for which I am extremely grateful.

Other early anaesthetic colleagues included Harry Wark and Victor Harrison, both in their ways superbly competent performers.

Of the Paediatric Cardiologists, Richard Hawker had trained in Johns Hopkins Hospital with Richard Rowe and also at Toronto Children's Hospital. He remained on Staff for over 50 years, maintained our Pathology collections and taught generations of aspiring physicians, and was the main instigator of our outreach clinics to regional centres, among numerous other initiatives. Chris Whight pioneered the essential new investigative tool of Echocardiology and much later migrated to Brisbane for another very successful career.

Gary Sholler was the first of our younger cardiologists, a great clinician with a flair for administration and development. As well as his clinical work, he eventually shouldered the heavy yoke of Director of the State's Paediatric Cardiology Services, an heroic effort to coordinate the usually warring services of the major Paediatric Hospitals in Sydney.

In 2018 he continued the struggle and seemed almost to savour it. [Gary finally despaired of the futile task of trying to create a unified NSW service and resigned in 2019 before the whole project was abandoned by the State Government some months later. In 2020 NSW Health, in its wisdom, decreed that there should be two separate Paediatric Cardiology/Cardiac Surgery Units for NSW].

Westmead

By the 1970s, Sydney's teaching hospitals and NSW's tertiary medical services had become hopelessly out of balance. The original University of Sydney Medical School hospitals were clustered around the inner city and lower North Shore, and even the University of New South Wales Medical School and its hospitals were largely confined to the Eastern Suburbs. With half the population of greater Sydney now living to the west of Parramatta, the State and Federal governments of the day were well justified in deciding to establish a major medical centre at Westmead. As expected, this attracted the usual naysayers, but construction went ahead and the new facility opened in 1978.

General Medical, Surgical and Obstetrical services were established first but Cardiology and Thoracic Surgery soon followed. My Children's Hospital colleague, David Johnson, was appointed Head of Cardiothoracic Surgery and began to perform chest operations. Johnson and Prof Miles Little, the Head of Surgery at the new hospital, invited me to join the staff. I agreed, on condition that I be excused from all administrative and medical-political duties. After prolonged wrangling at Ministerial level, we got the go-ahead to begin open-heart surgery.

John Uther had transferred from Prince Alfred to head up the medical Cardiology service; patients were flooding in.

We were fortunate to have as our anaesthetist Jeanne Collison, one of my trusted former colleagues from Prince Alfred, a very level-headed and effective person. Soon afterward Peter Klineberg returned after eight years in Pittsburgh, USA to join us.

I contributed one half day of operating a week plus some on-call work. Dave Johnson and I had soon performed 100 coronary operations with very low mortality, and with excellent graft patency proven by routine post-operative angiography [indicating a successful procedure].

Surgery for coronary disease and valvular heart disease was our main task. Uther and Johnson were keenly interested in investigation and surgical treatment of abnormal heart rhythms and they and their colleagues developed a major research focus on this topic. I left this demanding work to Johnson, while treating a growing number of adolescent and adult patients with congenital heart disease, some newly diagnosed and others who had been successfully operated on in infancy and childhood, grown to maturity, and were now in need of further surgery.

I enjoyed my continuing collaboration with David Johnson and my renewed exposure to coronary surgery. The only drawback was the geographical distance between Westmead and Camperdown, although my home was about equidistant from both. After a few years, my other commitments grew too demanding and my Westmead practice became largely confined to adult congenital heart disease.

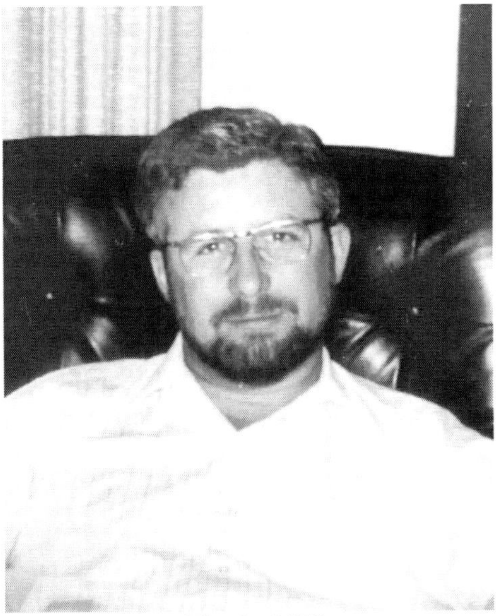

Tim in 1970

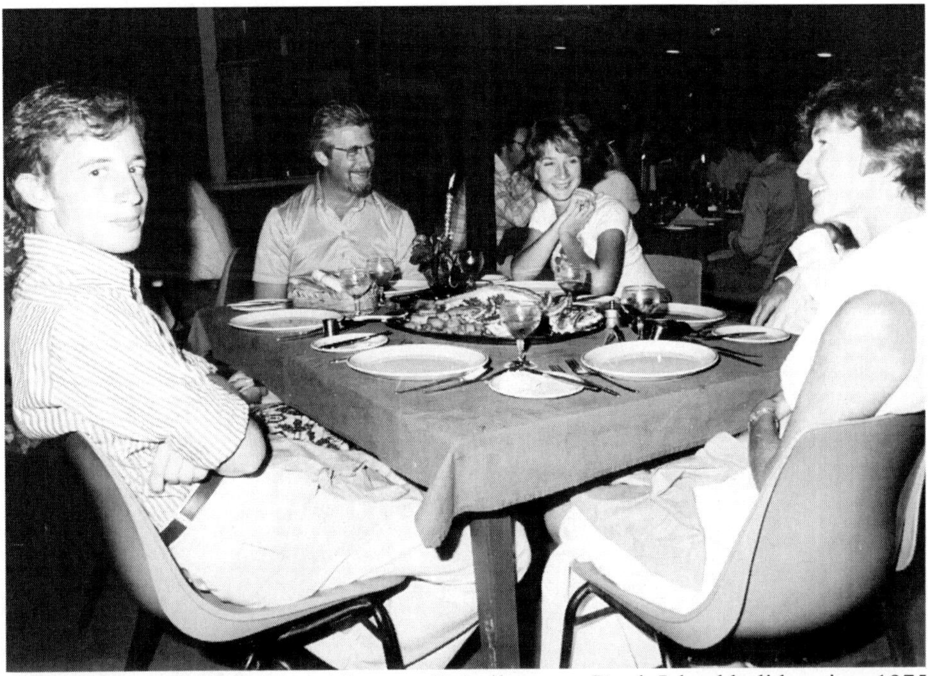

John Cartmill (left), Tim, Alison and Marilyn on a Dunk Island holiday circa 1975

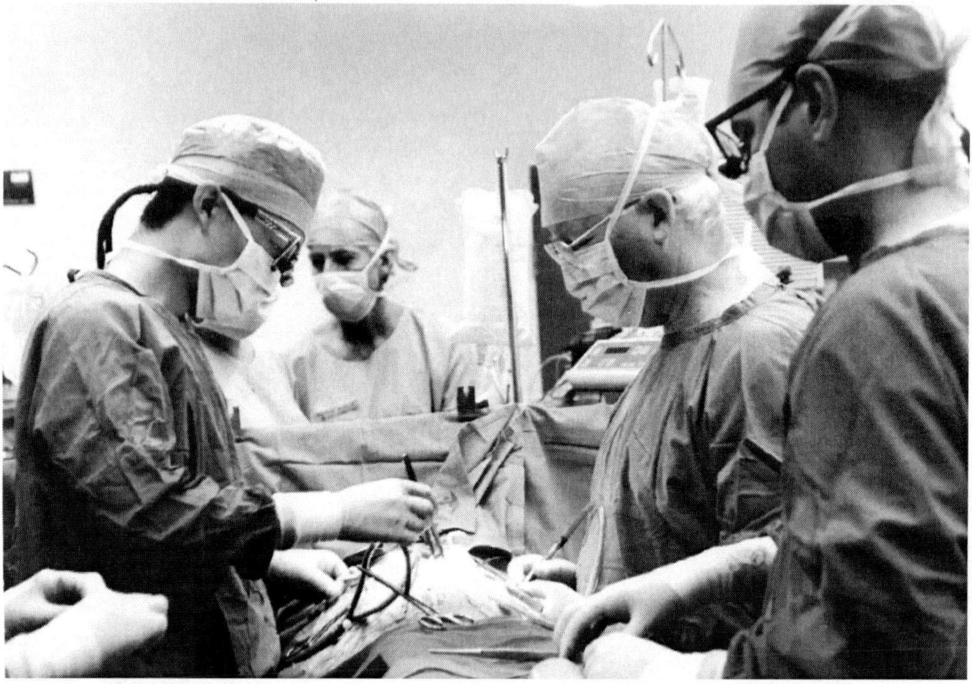

Tim (third from left) and colleagues with anaesthetist Harry Wark (second from left) circa 1980

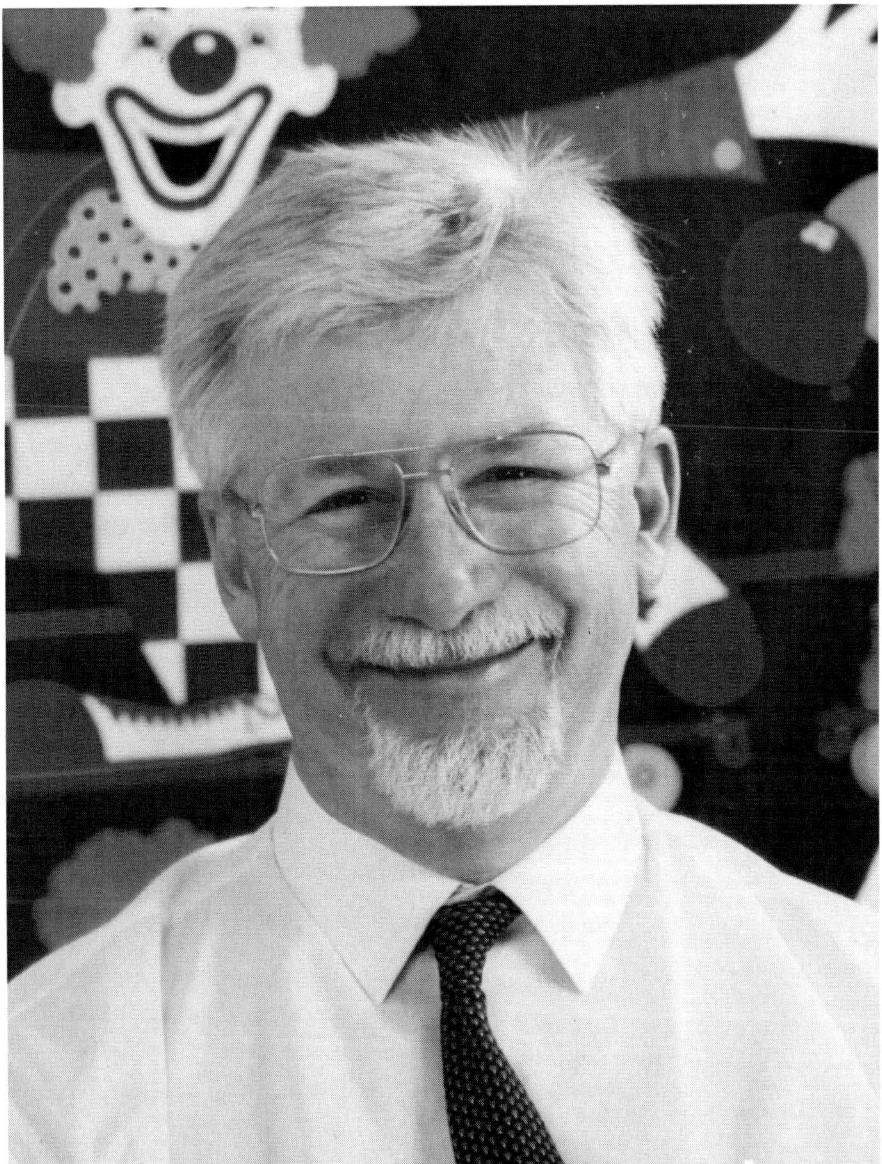

Tim circa 1997

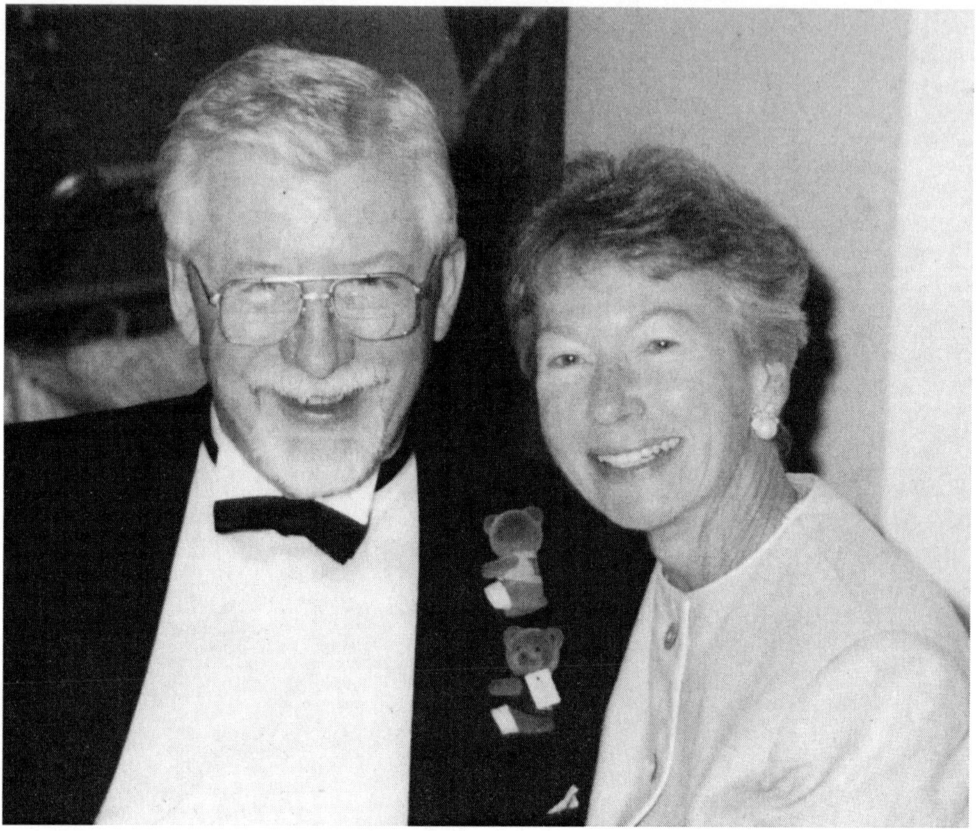

Tim and Marilyn circa 1988

Chapter 6: 'Third world' surgery

Cardiac surgery is hard at the best of times. To be successful and safe it requires preparation, teamwork, confidence and precision. To operate in a completely foreign environment is much harder. Alien languages and cultures, unfamiliar equipment, assistants of unknown competence and reliability, and above all, lack of many of the safety mechanisms which normally catch the latent errors; all these are likely pitfalls.

There is a case to be made for not operating away from the home base. Nevertheless, I enjoyed working in many developing countries, without having planned to do so. It proved to be challenging, yet intellectually and emotionally rewarding.

India

Around 1970, at the instigation of Rowan Nicks, Stanley John invited me to visit the Christian Medical College Hospital in Vellore, Tamil Nadu (Madras State), South India.

I sought the advice of Dr KM Cherian, a young Indian surgeon then training with us at Children's Hospital who had previously worked at CMC. Cherian helped to plot out an itinerary including several cardiac centres and some must-see tourist destinations, and I set off for the first of many daunting but enjoyable trips to India.

Stanley John met me at Madras and drove me to Vellore. This dry dusty inland market city is famed by some wits for having "a fort without soldiers, a river without water, and women without beauty". (The fort had police, not military, the river had been dammed upstream and was now dry, but the women looked fine to me.)

The Vellore Christian Mission had been founded by an American Missionary, Ida Hudder, who was inspired by the plight of women who were forbidden to seek help in childbirth from male doctors. Vellore has become a large medical facility including clinics, inpatient and outreach care, and hosts one of the best and most competitive medical schools in the country. Thoracic surgery had been established by an American, Dr Reeve Betts. Prof Gopinath had performed the first open heart operations in India there, before transferring to the All India Institute of Medical Sciences in Delhi. Stanley John was Gopinath's successor.

Stan is small framed, neat, punctiliously polite, dogmatic but with a touch of saintliness. He was well trained by Walt Lillehei in Minneapolis. Autocratic and demanding, he ran a tight ship. His wife, Dr Lily John, a general physician, was an Indian beauty, pleasant and friendly, and a very fine cook. They were a strong couple, and excellent hosts. Later on, it was our pleasure to care for them in return on their visits to Australia.

India is overwhelming. Everyone emphasises the heat and dust, the filth, the sights and sounds, the bustling crowds, the noise, the hubbub, the colour, the complexity, the smell. Not so many writers have witnessed it from the inside of Indian medical clinics or operating rooms.

Back in the 1970s there were just a few heart surgery centres to serve the needs of a population approaching one billion people. There was so much competition for so few resources in a society so generally short of everything, but so accustomed to struggle and striving. It was the most hectic marketplace imaginable.

The corridors of the clinic were packed with a throng of aspiring patients, pushing and shoving for attention in that particularly Indian way, superficially polite but surely insistent. Mothers and grannies held their children all day for a chance to see the man (occasionally a woman) in a white coat.

The doctors somehow maintained their equilibrium, judgement and polite attention through this pandemonium, day after hot sweaty day, and did their best to select patients who could be offered some medical or surgical help. Being India, there were abundant functionaries, servants, supervisors, and hangers-on to match the throng of potential customers. Paperwork was endless but there were plenty of clerks at hand to provide the service.

The operating rooms presented their own chaos. The surgeons were few and far between, seriously pressed for time, equipment, drugs, resources and everything else needed. Nurses and trainee assistant surgeons were in oversupply, each pushing for attention and kudos, all anxious for knowledge and advancement. This produced a peculiar style of operating in which there were many more assistants than necessary or ideal, all pressing into the scrum huddled around the patient, each trying desperately to contribute meaningfully and conspicuously. I have heard this style of operating aptly likened to "chooks feeding" as everybody pecks with one instrument or another at the operative field at any opportunity. This was accompanied by the usual high-pitched Indian babble. The fundamentals of the surgery are the same worldwide but here they were relying on very basic equipment and instruments that would long ago have been retired in the West. Every item was reused and adapted, washed and repurposed till it could not be possibly used another time – rather like the Indian cars.

At the end of this stifling high-energy day there was often some social occasion. This Indian version of the cocktail party, usually lubricated only by lukewarm fruit juice, has its own style, often held outdoors in the evening to alleviate the heat. The sexes were voluntarily segregated even more thoroughly than the Australian barbecue norms of the day. Simple spicy food was generously supplied. Here I first encountered the Indian coping skill of undermining everyone else, friend or foe, by belittling them in ways subtle and less subtle, denigrating them and their geographical, racial, religious or social status openly and in their hearing. This talent I characterised as stabbing people in the front.

Off to a restless hot sleep, to be awoken with bed-tea next morning and the whole process being replayed the next day. Intensive, overwhelming, sometimes threatening, ever-challenging, excellent, exciting, daunting – ultimately exhausting. And that was just the first port of call in Vellore. It was to be repeated in several other centres on that trip and on half a dozen more visits over the years. One thing about India, you don't forget it.

My old pupils, Dr M R S Menon and Dr John Tharian drove in from Trivandrum to join my farewell party. Tall in their long white calico lungis (sarongs or lap-laps), they cut a dash among the Vellore chaps who wore either Western style pants or shorter, patterned coloured lungis.

I clearly recall that road trip with Menon to the southwestern city of Trivandrum. Outside the towns there was not much car traffic on the narrow roads, but plenty of colourfully decorated trucks. The driving style was hyperactive and undisciplined but there were some conventions. The horn was in constant use, providing warnings to pedestrians, livestock, crows eating roadkill, even other trucks and cars. Cows took precedence over traffic, cars avoided trucks, cyclists often ran into the ditch for survival, and overtaking on the narrow roads was somehow accomplished without head-on collisions, usually. The farmers bent over their short-handled hoes to till the now dry rice fields, women dried the grain on the shoulder of the road and winnowed it by pitching it up into the breeze to separate the husk, and elderly pedestrians often carried an umbrella for shade as the sun grew ever hotter.

First stop was the famed Temple city of Madurai. Not one single temple, but a large city block, was crammed with immense stepped structures faced with sculptures and likenesses of the numerous Hindu gods. There was a sense of faded, sun-baked glory but the temples were in busy use. Worshippers aplenty attended their devotions or washed themselves in the huge temple tanks, great square well structures with giant steep steps leading down to the algal green holy water.

Rounding the tip of the Indian subcontinent, we skirted the mighty barrier of the Western Ghats, the mountain range running parallel with the western coast of the Peninsula. The arid lands of Tamil Nadu to the east gave way to the populous, fertile, green tropical state of Kerala. A land of beaches, tall waving coconut palms, steady rain fall, rice padis (paddies) and a bustling people. Many of them are Christians, considering themselves descended from the disciples of St Thomas. They are better educated on average than other Indians, and politically involved, having the distinction of having once installed the only freely elected Communist government in the world.

More consultations, more operations, more parties. Menon, Tharion and I visited KM Cherian's father, Mamen, a retired manager of a tea plantation in the mountains. We took tea beneath the glassy gaze of a huge tiger whose skin adorned the wall of his drawing room. Tigers had been a lethal pest in the mountains, killing livestock and villagers. Culling the rogues had been one of the Manager's tasks. Next day our long drive to the hills was interrupted when we broke our front suspension in a pothole. While our driver took the car to a village welder to be repaired, my hosts insisted I should try some todi, made of fermented coconut liquid. Not bad, and very popular in this non-prohibition state.

We pressed on into the afternoon, stopping for drinks with Mr Cherian's old fellow-planters at the former English Club in the mountains. Whisky was freely offered and the club President showed off the framed photos of former officials, waving his hand and announcing their causes of death. "Heart, liver, liver, heart, heart, et cetera". Hearty laughter all around! The last few miles took us to the mountain Game Reserve of Thekkady. We checked in and were taken after dark on a tour of the wildlife refuge, in hopes of seeing a tiger.

There were plenty of elephants, marvellous to see in the wild, but no tigers. I recollected the wall trophy at Mr Cherian's house.

Next major visit was with Prof N Gopinath in Delhi. As Stanley John's predecessor at Vellore, he had performed the first open heart operations in India and was now Professor of Surgery at the All India Institute of Medical Sciences in Delhi. Tall for an Indian, he was mature, wise, politically well-connected, a polymath who knew everyone and everything. A very inquisitive, intelligent, practical doer. As ever, the days were bustling and challenging, a non-stop round of consultations, conversations and presentations, interspersed with noisy operations.

Gopi was a friendly, kind and generous host. In contrast to the hectic days, we walked and talked in the calm and relative cool of the dawns in the surprisingly extensive parkland of Delhi, discussing many things.

As a side excursion he had arranged a weekend car trip to the must-see tourist cities of Agra and Jaipur. The Taj Mahal at Agra truly exceeds anyone's greatest expectations. So big, so symmetrical, so pure, so delicate, so glittering white in the dazzling light, so perfectly mirrored in the reflective pools of water.

Jaipur is another marvellous city to visit. Situated in the red plains of Rajasthan and built of pink stone, it rises above the desert. A trip on elephant-back up the long steep cutting to the Mughal Pink Palace was a highlight. The palace itself was a revelation, the size, the complexity of its mirrored rooms, the fretted stone privacy screens through which the ladies of the harem used peep out. Hospitality again was extraordinary as Gopinath had mobilised all his contacts in this city to honour me with a generous dinner.

On the next weekend I flew to Srinagar, Capital of Kashmir. Ever since the partition of India there has been serious tension between India and Pakistan over this truly beautiful part of the world in the foothills of the Himalaya. There was no active fighting at the time of my visit. My first lodging was one of hundreds of houseboats on the still, hyacinth-covered waters of the lake, served by gondola-like punts, poled by cheerful fellows selling flowers, food and every kind of treat. Ashore, the derelict rose gardens of a former palace barely survived.

Next day's trip was by car, high into the mountains to the former hill station of Gulmarg. Road workers squatted on the narrow roads, reducing big rocks to gravel size by knapping them with a handheld hammer. Before dinner I had time to climb behind the former English Club building beside the famed golf course, said to be the World's highest, puffing from the 3,000m altitude, to look up to the 8,000m snow topped Himalayan mass of Nanga Parbat beyond. It was a real privilege to have seen this sublime place while it was not marred by hot military conflict.

This first trip to India left impressions which have never faded, lifelong friendships, a hugely expanded appreciation of history and alien cultures and religions, and admiration for the spirit of the Indian people who thrive in their way. Although poor in financial terms, they navigate their difficulties in their own style.

Malaysia

In 1977 Rowan Nicks invited me to join him for a couple of weeks in Kuala Lumpur, where he was acting as locum for the recently departed Professor of Surgery at the University Medical Centre. The cardiac surgery was being performed by Dr Huat-Seong Saw, a very bright young Chinese Malaysian who had recently returned from working with Frank Spencer in New York. Rowan thought that Saw and I would get on well together and we did.

Kuala Lumpur was an interesting place at that time. Having separated from Singapore about a dozen years earlier, Malaysia was beginning to hit its stride politically and economically. There were still considerable political tensions and some recent violent riots as the Muslim native Malays pushed back against the political and commercial dominance of the Chinese. This ongoing unrest has led to the departure of many Chinese Malaysians to Singapore and elsewhere as they see little future for their children in the face of the Bhumiputera movement, an Affirmative Action policy which in effect gives preference to Malays in every field of politics, leadership, and academia.

I stayed with Rowan in his small apartment on campus and he was a kind and generous host. The flat was airy and shaded by coconut palms, complete with ever-chattering monkeys.

I operated a bit and talked a lot with Saw, and Rowan and I participated in the general teaching rounds at the University Hospital. After work, Rowan and I generally drove to the Officers' Club for a swim.

The local medical students were, like most medical students everywhere, a delight – keen, intelligent, friendly and hospitable. They liked to include Rowan and me in their evening outings in which they enjoyed Hindi movies, prodigious eating at the street stalls, and plenty of friendly conversation.

One weekend we drove north to the island of Penang where we stayed at the old Eastern and Oriental Hotel.

Rowan and I planned to return to Australia to attend the 50th anniversary Jubilee celebrations of the Royal Australasian College of Surgeons in Melbourne. Our trip was interrupted at Singapore airport where we were held up for a few days by an air traffic controllers' strike in Australia. The old Changi Airport Terminal was not a very comfortable place in which to wait out the delay.

I have been back to Malaysia several times. On one occasion Marilyn and I went for a holiday, while attending surgery conferences in Kuala Lumpur and Penang. This time we stayed at the University guest quarters and later drove ourselves around much of the peninsula of Malaysia. The less-developed East Coast was best. Forty years later we recall fondly our chicken-rice lunches eaten under a tin-roofed shack at truck stops on the road north, with chickens and cats around our feet. Another treat was to see a man managing a tame monkey which climbed the tall palms and tossed ripe coconuts to the ground at his command.

On a later visit I worked for a few days at the new University Kebangsaan Hospital in Kuala Lumpur city, accompanied by John Overton. We demonstrated our Paediatric Cardiac Surgery techniques using profound hypothermia. I had to leave Overton to help care for a couple of the slowly recovering patients while I flew to Singapore to join Marilyn. We were staying at the Australian High Commissioner's residence with Alison's in-laws, Walter and Norma Handmer, for a few days while I attended yet another College meeting in Singapore. To see the city as the guest of a diplomat was a rare treat. In that steamy heat, to be chauffeured around in the High Commissioner's limo with a flagpole on the front was true bliss. The icing on the cake was a phone call from John Overton a day or two later telling me that all the patients had made an excellent recovery.

The politics of the beautiful country of Malaysia are still uneasy but there is no gainsaying its tremendous progress since those times, with the increased prosperity, extraordinary building and general economic growth.

Dr HS Saw later migrated to become the outstanding cardiac surgeon at the private Queen Elizabeth Hospital in Singapore.

China

Victor Chang was an attractive fellow, intelligent, clever, diligent, competent, charming, entrepreneurial and persuasive. I readily agreed to accompany him and Mark Shanahan on a trip to China, soon after it began opening up to the rest of the world in about 1983.

Familiar with the benefits of public relations, it was no surprise that he felt the need to accompany us with a professional documentary film making team of cinematographer, director, and director's gofer.

First stop was Hong Kong. We landed late in the evening and joined Victor's father for a fine Chinese feast. Where better to have it? Chang Senior was a kind host although he spoke little English, despite having lived for some years in Australia.

Next day we set out for Beijing, formerly Peking. As we boarded the CAC aircraft Victor pronounced, correctly, "From here on everything is second-class", referring to accommodation, travel facilities and so forth. Beijing had not yet developed much beyond the closed Communist era. The ten-lane highway from the airport had almost no cars but innumerable bicycles. Some new building was going on and we stayed the first few nights in a new development area, before moving downtown to a more fitting establishment. There was little sign of modernisation of the society. Men and women all still wore khaki or blue quilted Mao suits and there was no sign of consumer goods, apart from the duty-free stuff in the tourist store.

The hospital was massive and busy. Victor, Mark and I did a few operations with satisfactory results. The operating rooms were primitive. After scrubbing up with harsh brushes and caustic soap we still had to immerse our hands and forearms in deep jars of alcohol because the water supply to the operating rooms was not sterile. I well remember the sting of the scratches from the brushing.

Victor showed us around the attractions of the central city including Red Square and the Emperor's Palace. On a spare day we took the mandatory bus trip to the Great Wall. It is as great as anyone could expect. The portion we saw has been well restored and we climbed a fair distance along it up one of the hills. The tremendous structure snakes away to the horizon, zig-zagging to maintain its course along the ridgelines.

Somewhat surprisingly, there were still temples to be seen along the way, and the ones we visited were crowded with supplicants recording their hopes and fears by leaving little twists of paper in niches in the walls.

Next stop was Guangzhou, formerly Canton, on the Pearl River far to the south. In clear contrast with Beijing, many of the people, especially the young, wore colourful Western clothing, with denim jeans being popular. Street markets sold many consumer goods. Here I actually saw and heard my first "ghetto blaster". Canton was well ahead of me in audio fashion.

At the Medical Centre, Victor had a couple of interesting commercial projects afoot. One was the manufacture of artificial heart valves using a popular American design but assembling them out of Patent and free of American Standards and liability provisions, and hence at a fraction of the international price. This made them feasible in the large potential markets of China and India.

The second project involved pig valves, which were processed for human surgery in a high-quality aseptic environment. The Chinese technicians were superb at this needlework, stitching the valve into a supporting sewing ring with perfect technique.

In the room next to this high-tech clean manufacturing facility was a Dispensary devoted to traditional Chinese medicines, which are still popular and freely used. The juxtaposition of pickled snakes next door to the space-age germfree room was startling.

A fast ferry trip down the Pearl River returned us to Hong Kong, thence to our flight to Sydney to complete a very interesting trip.

Vanuatu

Republic of Vanuatu
Memorandum
26th October 1992

From: Hospital Management Team
To: All Doctors & All Head of Sections and Staff
Subject: Time Change

We have been directed the new time change.

Please note that really there should be no disruptions of timetables. Eg: New Time 8:30 AM is the same as old-time 7:30 AM.

So even if you do not change your watch and you keep to the old time you will still be following the new time, bearing in mind of course that you are one hour behind of new time.

If the new times confuses our current timetables. Please leave them as they are and keep to the old-time.

Dr SB, A/Medical Superintendent, VCH

This little gem of bureaucratese graced the noticeboard of the General Hospital at Vanuatu. On reflection, it is not the most obscure pronouncement I have read on daylight saving, or medical administration.

Marilyn and I had been recruited for the Heart Surgery outreach trip to Vanuatu. Russell Lee, an Intensive Care Nurse at the Seventh Day Adventist Hospital, "The San", at Wahroonga in Sydney had, while visiting his Missionary parents in Tonga, conceived the idea of bringing highly specialised services to the Pacific Islands, which at that time had no chance of providing them for themselves, with Fiji the largest island group, with about one million people.

Vanuatu, formerly known as the New Hebrides and administered as a condominium by France and Great Britain, had some 200,000 people occupying an archipelago scattered over more than 1,000 km in the Southwest

Pacific. Remnants of the bilingual administration persisted. Most government services were somehow duplicated by language and tradition. Local malefactors were said to prefer the French jail because the food was much better.

At their first visit, to Tonga, the "Sanatorium" team had performed mostly heart valve surgery but recognised that there was an overwhelming need for treatment of children with congenital heart disease. My old friend and former pupil Peter Brady asked me to join a second visit, to Vanuatu.

Russell Lee and his supporters had set up a sound team structure, based on the Seventh Day charity the Adventist Development and Relief Agency (ADRA). Support was recruited from far and wide. Many hospitals donated out-of-date or unused equipment, and various medical supply companies gave equipment or other help in kind. Nurses, medical staff, technicians and other volunteers, mostly from Melbourne and Sydney, donated their time and airfares, and the whole expedition was managed quite professionally.

One Sunday, many of the team mustered at the Sanatorium Hospital in Fox Valley Road and sorted through equipment, dressings, drugs and any other things that we might find useful, and prepared them for packing and airfreight to the island.

We were preceded by a technical team who flew into the Capital, Port Vila, on the island of Efate. Their task was to improve the technical facilities of the old hospital sufficiently for our work. A left-over from World War II, the faded huts of the hospital were built in two or three parallel rows, connected by open outdoor walkways sheltered by a fibro roof. Each hut held one Nightingale pattern ward, with simple bedsteads close together in a dormitory layout. Patients were usually surrounded by relatives who provided most of their care and feeding.

The single operating room hut was small and cramped. Walls and ceilings were mouldy from the oppressive humid heat. A former member of the medical staff had dealt with the unsightly mould by liberally spraying ceilings, walls and anything else within reach with chlorine bleach from a knapsack spray. This temporarily suppressed the mould but permanently rusted fast the mechanisms and casters of the operating table and the adjustable hinges of the light. Our team of engineers beefed up the electrical wiring and medical gas supplies to the Operating Theatre and a couple of ward beds.

Our Paediatric team had arranged for Gary Sholler, Paediatric Cardiologist from Sydney's Royal Alexandra Hospital for Children, supported by an echocardiography technician, to precede us and assess the many potential candidates for surgery. Gary winnowed the field to those he considered most likely to benefit from an operation without presenting excessive surgical risk, selecting more patients for us than we could possibly have treated. This was sensible; not all of them turned up. Some from outer islands could not come because "the diesel for the motor launch had run out". A few more absconded before surgery.

Our team members were lodged in one of the two resort hotels which had donated rooms. This generous gift, along with free meals from many of the restaurants on the island, constituted most of the local contribution. The hospital lent us an ancient Pajero for our local transport.

Our first day was taken up by an intensive clinical session in which we reviewed Gary's chosen cases and assembled a tentative operating list. We intentionally selected fairly simple cases which were unlikely to fail; there was no point in jeopardising the program at its beginning. We were also relying on rapid postoperative recoveries so our limited resources could handle a reasonable number of patients.

Anaesthetists, David Baines from the Children's Hospital and John Holmes from the Royal North Shore Hospital, and the scrub nurses, largely from the San and Royal Children's Hospital in Melbourne, readied their equipment and instruments. The Perfusionists, from a group who provided Heart Lung Perfusion services for some of the major Melbourne private hospitals, had cobbled together a simple portable Heart-Lung machine.

Brady and I managed two open heart operations most days, which is not bad going in unfamiliar territory with an unaccustomed team. Peter would operate on the adults while I took care of the children. My assistant was the current Cardiac Surgery Registrar from Children's Hospital, Dr Suresh Rao. Postoperative nursing was handled faultlessly by the volunteers, including three of our most senior nurses from Camperdown Children's Hospital and more from Melbourne's Royal Children's, with several others from The Adventist Hospital. The surgery went well, and we usually finished in good time to enjoy some liquid team building and good fellowship in the resort bar, later eating either in the hotel or at one of the island's fine restaurants.

It was an intensive two weeks of hard work. The basic principles of open-heart surgery, with which I had grown up 30 and more years earlier, worked well without needing to rely on elaborate equipment or techniques. Post-operative care, similarly, needed to be kept simple and basic because we lacked anything other than essential monitors, respirators, and drugs. Most heartening was the easy professionalism and good spirit which everybody brought to the project. Well trained and highly motivated people easily coalesce into effective teams. Each of us learned a lot from our new colleagues; a bonus.

Most importantly, all the patients did well and recovered rapidly, establishing beyond doubt that Paediatric Cardiac Surgery could be performed successfully under these conditions. The Melanesian children were charming and undemanding, the parents grateful, and the island population supportive and friendly.

It was not all work. One weekend a group of us took a bus tour around the island. Highlights included swimming off pristine beaches and snorkelling over the coral. At the far western end of the island, sheltered from the sun by the tall coconut palms, we visited the area in which the writer James Michener had lived while writing "Tales of the South Pacific". Nearer to the capital, Port Vila, were huge outcrops of the kudzu vine which had been used by the Americans during the War to camouflage their equipment. Maybe the weed will never be controlled. Though most of the island is hilly and covered in jungle or coconut glades, some of the area closer to town is relatively flat and suitable for grazing and farming.

A group of us flew the 40 minutes by Britton-Norman Islander aircraft south to the enchanted island of Tanna. This smaller island is dominated by its active volcano, Yasur. Tanna is far less sophisticated than Efate, mostly a subsistence economy supported by fishing and yam, coconut and pig farming. The main drawback of this island paradise is the prevalence of the "malignant", often fatal, form of malaria caused by the mosquito-borne parasite Plasmodium falciparum.

Marilyn and I had been assigned lodgings at White Grass resort, a small cluster of woven palm frond huts surrounding a common dining area and bar, right on the edge of the ocean. Once we had eliminated most of the ants which fell copiously from the thatch of the roof onto our bedding, we were comfortable enough and I thought it would be a good place to return to someday, to write The Novel and enjoy a cold beer at sunset.

Our main tourist activity was the obligatory circuit of the island. Our guide and jeep driver took us ever higher through the sterile lava fields in the lee of the volcano, stopping about a hundred metres from the summit. From there we scrambled up to the unguarded rim, where we looked down into the swirling molten rock of the caldera, surrounded by stinking sulphur fumes, and probably lucky not to be struck by some of the rocks continuously being flung into the sky. In hindsight, it was not a very intelligent place to be.

Having survived the volcano, we stopped at a Kastom village to see their dances and activities. (Kastom is the local Bislama language word embracing culture and religion.) The village consists of little huts of woven palm fronds with palm thatch roofs. Enclosures for the pigs are defined by trenches which separate the animals from the yam gardens.

The tribal dancing was most spectacular. The men were sturdy and muscular, their black skins gleaming with sweat, and totally naked apart from their penis gourds. Women were also strong and fit looking, topless, their lower body partly covered by “arse grass”, or grass skirts. Unfortunately, it is fairly common for these skirts to catch fire. The frenzied tempo of the dancing shakes the ground and raises the dust from their stamping feet.

Another part of the “Kastom” of these people is the cargo cult which worships John Frum. There are several theories about the origin of this cult, but a common theme is that it arose from the arrival of the American forces in World War II who came in their aeroplanes from the sky, bringing “cargo” of vehicles and motorcycles, cigarettes, candy and tinned food. When the tall white-skinned uniformed strangers were asked who they were, their leaders said: “I'm John frum America”. Whatever the origin, the belief persists and is celebrated at an annual ceremony in which the local tribe erects bamboo flagpoles and make-believe radio antennae, marches back and forth, and tries once more to call down the cargo from the sky. Possibly related is the belief that the Duke of Edinburgh is some kind of white God. During his Royal visits to the island the natives saw this tall white-faced uniformed man accompanying his wife, the Queen, both of them treated with such obvious deference.

This successful and highly gratifying expedition to Vanuatu set the pattern for another half dozen trips over the next several years. Using a similar team structure but increasing sophistication of equipment and organisation, we made several visits to Fiji and one further trip to Vanuatu.

Fiji

The Fiji island group is larger than Vanuatu and has about one million people. Access is easy through the international airport at Nadi. Having once flown from Nadi on the West coast to Suva in the east in a violent and turbulent electrical storm, in a small aircraft with the jungle visible through holes in its floor, we usually arranged to stay overnight in the Nadi area then drive a rented car around the southern coast of the island to our destination.

The town of Suva is bustling, with mainly Melanesian and Indian people, and is a lively tourist area in its own right. On our first visit the hospital was a typical old colonial institution without much sophistication. Subsequently a modern hospital block built by the Japanese was much more convenient.

The Adventist outreach activities later became associated with a program initiated by the Australian Government's Department of Foreign Affairs. Having supported several individual surgical programs in the Pacific Islands, especially Plastic Surgery and Ophthalmic surgery, the Australian Government tasked the Royal Australasian College of Surgeons to report on possible reorganisation and amalgamation of these efforts.

I was nominated by the College, of which I was then a Council member, to join Ross Naylor, a Foreign Aid expert, to evaluate all these DFAT programs. Ross and I travelled to Vanuatu, Fiji and Tonga and recommended a scheme of future management.

Out of this grew the Pacific Island Project funded largely by the Australian Government and administered through the Royal Australasian College of Surgeons. This made for more predictable funding and secured more up-to-date equipment. The Adventist Outreach program maintained its volunteer professional characteristics, in which the medical and nursing staff volunteered their time, airfares and professional services pro bono.

With my retirement from practice in Australia in 1997 I ceased all further involvement with these programs. They have grown and prospered, with many more expeditions, including Fiji, Papua New Guinea, Tonga, Rwanda, Nepal, Myanmar, the Philippines, Solomon Islands, China, Cambodia, Tanzania and even Mongolia. The physicians, surgeons, anaesthetists, perfusionists, nurses and others who have supported this work have my greatest admiration.

My friend David Baines has recently retired after 20 trips and counts this as one of the most satisfying activities of his career. Russell Lee, now AO, the visionary nurse whose inspiration started it all, continues as Director in its present incarnation called Open Heart International.

It has been difficult to transfer these highly specialised skills of cardiac surgery to the doctors in the small communities. However, Graham Nunn, after several trips to Papua and New Guinea taught local surgeons to perform some of the simpler operations.

Mongolia

This story begins with a little child who was sent to Sydney for surgery in 1995. Ishigul, a two year old Mongolian girl, had been born with the complex congenital heart defect of atrioventricular septal defect (in which the central part of the heart fails to develop properly, with the result that large parts of the atrial and ventricular septa and many of the components of the mitral and tricuspid valves are missing). A group of Rotarians from the Wahroongah Club who happened to be in the Capital of Ulaanbaatar learned of her plight and arranged for Ishigul, accompanied by her father, to come to Sydney for surgery. In view of the complexity of her problem, the doctors at Wahroonga wisely decided to refer her for diagnosis and treatment at the Children's Hospital in Camperdown. With the detailed diagnosis established by our cardiologists,

I performed corrective surgery and she was later transferred back to the Adventist hospital for recuperation. She made a good recovery and her policeman father was delighted.

A couple of years later Alan Gale mobilised an Outreach team for an expedition to the Mongolian capital with a view to introducing some Western techniques there. We understood that they had been doing open-heart surgery but the results had not been ideal.

Gale thought it appropriate to document this trip by a video production, so the usual volunteer nurses, doctors and perfusionists were accompanied by a television production team. Our first stop was Beijing, where we spent a day or two in the usual tourist pursuits before flying to Xian to see the recently unearthed "terracotta warriors". These realistic life-sized pottery soldiers are thought to have been made for burial with some ancient ruler to guard him in the afterlife. They are an extraordinary sight, now housed under a giant awning to protect them from the worst of the weather.

We flew across the Gobi Desert to Ulaanbaatar before seemingly landing in the municipal tip, so dense was the trash blowing around in the cold dusty wind. Until recently Outer Mongolia had been garrisoned by about one million Soviet troops who had spent many decades confronting the Chinese across the border. The Russians' rapid departure left the economy destitute and the structures ramshackle. It was the first city in which I had seen all the indoor heating provided by a centralised boiler house connected with a large red-lagged steam pipe to the individual buildings. Our hotel, the cleverly named Genghis Khan, was one of the few modern buildings in the centre of town. Meals were simple. As we had difficulty with the language it was safest to rely on fried eggs for breakfast and some kind of stewed meat of doubtful origin for dinner, or maybe fish (now where might that have come from?)

The hospital was Soviet style and very basic. Everything was in desperately short supply. Surgical instruments were sterilised by heaping them in a hand basin, dousing them in methylated spirits, and setting fire to them. Monitoring equipment was of the typical sturdy Soviet style but it worked. The heart-lung machine was an early Japanese model I think, very heavy and difficult to control. They relied on a reusable stainless steel bubble oxygenator device. Not surprisingly, they had little confidence in this equipment and preferred to use hypothermia with inflow occlusion, with predictably imperfect repairs. The electrical safety was terrifying, with naked earth wires, joined by twisting their bare ends together, snaking across the sopping wet floors.

We had a strong medical team. Chris Whight, an old Paediatric Cardiologist friend from Brisbane, worked tirelessly with his echocardiography technician to try to inculcate some of his skill and knowledge to their local counterparts. David Cole, a Cardiologist from Canberra, similarly taught all he could of the principles and practice of coronary angiography to the cardiologists. Anaesthetist Peter Lindburgh managed the anaesthesia while Peter Klineberg concentrated on perfusion, using the local, very basic, pump chassis with the disposable oxygenators which we had brought with us.

Alan Gale achieved his ambition of performing the first coronary bypass graft operation in Mongolia. I thought it prudent to avoid complex surgery in that primitive setting but agreed to perform a palliative Blalock shunt operation on a very blue child with tetralogy of Fallot. I judged that this would have the best chance of success with predictable improvement in the child's condition, and would do no harm.

The procedure did not go to plan as Dr Lindburgh had great difficulty inducing anaesthesia in this already critically hypoxic patient. Instead of going to sleep and breathing more steadily with induction of anaesthesia, the child struggled and became more and more agitated. Her anaesthetist realised that something was not right and finally disconnected the tubing and took a sniff to check what was being inhaled. To his horror he found that the anaesthetic machine had been filled from an old Halothane anaesthetic agent bottle which now contained methylated spirit. Empty glass bottles were so precious that they could not be discarded. Once Peter had replaced the alcohol with the correct agent, anaesthesia was established and there was no more trouble. The operation was uneventful and the result about as good as we could have expected. I rate that as one of the slickest recoveries from near disaster I have ever seen an anaesthetist perform.

As well as our surgery, we conducted clinics and gave lectures to the hospital staff. Social engagements were friendly and hospitable, often including a certain amount of drinking. At a farewell ceremony we were entertained by Mongolian music and folk dancing, numerous speeches, and the presentation of an Award to Alan Gale. After lengthy felicitations he was draped in an elaborate embroidered gown and concluded the ceremony by drinking a large ceremonial bowl of fermented mare's milk. It was a heroic performance; it is always nice to be thanked.

On a weekend we took a long bus trip westward from the capital, climbing through the grazing lands towards heavily wooded mountains. Although poor and harsh it is a most beautiful part of the world. The local people in the warmer months live in easily demountable and transportable circular tents so that they may follow their herds on the upland pastures. These tents, called gurs, are essentially the same as what we usually call yurts. A light wooden framework supports the insulated felt walls. Entry is through a low doorway on the leeward side, a small fire burns in the centre with smoke partly escaping through a central hole in the roof. Bedding is arranged around the periphery with females on one side and males on the other. Hospitality is generous and mostly consists of vodka. Interestingly, living in these gurs is also encouraged within the city limits where each family is assigned their own individual block on which to erect it.

It was a marvellous trip to this little-known part of the world. We were shown great hospitality and some of the local medical staff were keen to learn from us. It was frustrating not to have been able to do more advanced surgery.

One highlight was to meet again our original patient, Ishigul, now five years old, and her policeman father who had been promoted since his trip to Australia. The little girl was bright and active. Chris Whight examined the heart with echocardiography and found that my repair was working very well. We paid a social visit to the whole family in their gur.

Ukraine in 1992, 2001, 2011

Sometimes great things develop unexpectedly. The 1986 Chernobyl nuclear reactor accident provided a surprising example. A year or so after the disaster, a group of Canberra Rotarians led by Jack Olssen visited Kyiv, Ukraine, to arrange for a group of radiation affected children to come to Australia for a respite exchange. During his visit to Kyiv, Olssen was made aware of numerous babies and children who were in need of surgical treatment for congenital heart diseases. There was an active Heart Institute, but it was not dealing with complex defects in children.

With the cooperation of our general superintendent, Dr John Yu, Olssen arranged for four young doctors from the Amosov Institute, Kyiv, to visit Royal Alexandra Hospital for Children in Camperdown for about three months, housing them in the Residents' quarters.

The visitors were supported by the Rotary Club organisation and by members of the Ukrainian community in Sydney. These Ukrainian expats, mainly refugees from the post-war era, had settled successfully in Sydney. Led by Strathfield GP Christina Bilinsky, they later raised money to provide equipment for this new heart surgery venture in Kyiv.

We greeted the team with some apprehension, as the Cold War was only receding after the collapse of the Soviet Union, and our knowledge of Ukraine was extremely sketchy.

Ukraine is larger than most European countries, and composed mostly of flat fertile agricultural country, crossed from north to south by three major rivers
of which the largest is the Dneiper. In about 900 CE the area was colonised by Vikings using the river as a trade route from the Baltic towards the Black Sea. The ruler Volodomyr the Great converted to Christianity. Reportedly he chose the Greek Orthodox religion after rejecting Judaism because he was fond of pork, Roman Catholicism because he did not care for celibacy, and Islam because he was not attracted by adult circumcision. He forcibly baptised the whole Kyiv town populace in the waters of the great river. The resulting Kyiv Rus civilisation became a dominant power and ruled a wide surrounding area for about 250 years. They were overrun by Mongols from the east and later

carved up time and again from various directions by Poland, Russia, Prussia, Austria, and Lithuania. Eventually Catherine the Great of Russia reached Crimea in 1854. The Crimean War was fought as the British, French and Ottomans tried to deny Russian access to a warm water port on the Black Sea.

The 20th Century did not go well. After the 1917 Russian Revolution and a brief period of independence and then civil war, the victory of the Red Army resulted in the incorporation of Ukraine territory into the USSR. Ukraine continued its historic role as a food bowl under rural collectivisation and Russian repression. After a terrible famine in the 1930s, World War II was also disastrous for Ukraine when the Nazis invaded via the western part adjoining Poland. Various dissidents, who had been stirring up trouble against the Russians, found it expedient to collaborate with the Nazis. As a result, Ukrainians were fighting Ukrainians and Russians. These tensions persisted after Ukraine became independent of Russia after the fall of the Soviet Union in 1991. These divisions remain, with much of Western Ukraine looking towards Europe and influenced, like Poland, by Roman Catholicism, while the industrialised Eastern region remains largely faithful to Russia and Greek orthodox religion. Kyiv sits in the middle and its politics remain unstable, allegedly corrupt, and baffling to an onlooker.

Returning to our Ukrainian visitors in Camperdown: the leader, surgeon Ilya Yemets, was a very bright, energetic young man, who at that stage had very little English. His anaesthetist, a Russian named Alexander Masur, was quite fluent. Paediatric cardiologist Alex Perepeka had some English and was a very charming fellow. The fourth member of the team was a heart-lung machine expert, who mostly dealt with our chief technician at the time, Paul Bernhardt. As a group, the Ukrainians were serious, conscientious, and probably as wary of us as we were guarded about them. Masur in particular had a disconcerting habit of taking extensive notes in a little red book. Some of the hospital wits suggested he was KGB.

In the northern hemisphere summer of 1992, I was invited to visit Kyiv for about 10 days. Flying via Frankfurt, I arrived at Kyiv to be greeted by Ilya and spirited through customs by his contacts. He drove me into town along a broken and deserted highway between rows of identical precast concrete apartment blocks, across the mighty Dneiper River, past the gigantic triumphal hilltop statue of a heroic Soviet warrior, and established me in an old, thin-walled, timber panelled hotel.

Conditions were dire. In the short period since the fall of the USSR, Ukraine had emerged as a poor but independent state. The cobbled streets were almost free of traffic and the only cars were Ladas of various ages. Some shops were open but there was nothing in them to buy. There was no real money, only photocopied "coupons". Most of the people were shabby and dour.

There followed a hectic period of work and play. First stop the next morning was the Amosov Cardiac Institute, another gloomy concrete pile, shabbily constructed and charmless with the exception of the nicely panelled Director's office in the front hall. There I met the Chief, Academician Knyshov, and later Professor Amosov, renowned pioneer Soviet cardiac surgeon. Although in his 80s, he came to work most days and pottered about. They treat retired professors with a bit more respect there.

I soon reacquainted myself with the Sydney team and we settled into the usual helter-skelter of case reviews, consultations with patients and parents, and in due course some operations. Ilya's paediatric team, young, keen, and clearly trying to strike in a new direction, appeared to be held at arm's length by the rest of the medical and surgical staff. The senior staff seemed content to plod along, performing perhaps one straightforward operation each before calling it a day. It was a strange contrast with the culture of every cardiac surgery outfit I had seen, where, in spite of individual differences, nearly all the staff were keen for work, thirsty for challenge, and mostly bustling with energy.

The operating rooms were spartan. The Russian style equipment looked clunky but worked well enough. The surgery team was excellent with the perfusionists working efficiently and safely and the nurses diligent and skilful. Most impressive was the senior scrub nurse, Lyudmilla, who had everything under control.

Ilya and I performed several operations together. Towards the end of this stay I performed an arterial switch operation for a baby with transposition of the great arteries. This is a demanding procedure and can only be done with modern equipment including special double-ended polypropylene sutures. [These very fine sutures are manufactured with the eyeless needles pre-attached to either end, "swaged on", so they can be passed without damage to the delicate blood vessels]. One of my operating habits had been to snap these needles

off to save a few seconds before tying the knot. Lyudmilla was quick to show her displeasure at this wasteful and thoughtless behaviour. She instead would retrieve the intact ends of the sutures, so they could be tied together and reused after re-sterilisation — a small illustration of the economic difficulties under which they functioned.

The patients did well, much to the credit of Dr Alex Masur who not only anaesthetised the children but where necessary stayed with them overnight to ensure detailed care.

Social activities were many and testing. At weekends we had several expeditions out of town. One was a drizzly visit to a farm area on which historical farm buildings from all over Ukraine had been re-erected as a museum. Reminiscent in some ways of the old timber barns and some of the equipment from my childhood. Always these expeditions were an excuse for a picnic of some kind, accompanied by a good deal of hard liquor. Food was simple. It was springtime so there was a variety of fresh salads, but not much meat, with the exception of slabs of pork fat and crackling. This I learned much later was a traditional Ukrainian delicacy called salo.

Another memorable expedition was a weekend picnic on an island within the Dneiper River, accessed on a very shaky boat. While the guests ran about and played with a football the boat's skipper barbecued some bits of pork on skewers. This captain was a tough guy: as he went about his work in shirtsleeves I was swaddled in my own underwear, all the sweaters I could lay hands on, and an outer layer of the padded Soviet military gear. I could not remember ever being so cold.

The hectic visit came to an end and we had a great farewell party in the conference room of my hotel. My contribution was a splendid fruitcake which Marilyn had baked in anticipation. That cake was well received and heartily accompanied by Georgian Cognac and Russian vodka.

On return to Australia, I had the honour of addressing the Press Club in Canberra about this program, and received a Paul Harris Rotary Club medal for my pains.

A year or two later, Ilya returned to Sydney for a longer visit of about six months, this time accompanied by a surgical assistant. His English was now quite good, and his knowledge rapidly improving. Around this time, he also spent extensive periods in Melbourne, Toronto, and Paris, thirstily acquiring the latest expertise from leading world centres.

Second Kyiv visit, 2001

In 2001, while I was nearing the end of my stay in Abu Dhabi, I was again invited to Kyiv, approximately nine years after the original trip. This time I flew in via Zürich, across the seemingly never-ending farmlands and villages of Switzerland, Austria, and the southern part of Germany, landing in the midst of the 10th anniversary celebration of Ukraine's independence from USSR.

Things had looked up. The airport terminal was bigger and smarter. Ilya's old Lada had been upgraded to a smart new Opel people mover. My accommodation was a well-furnished flat in the centre of town owned by one of Ilya's lawyer friends and set up with an office and sitting room, a small kitchen and bedroom and bathroom.

The city itself had largely come back to life with restoration of many of the public buildings, repair of the streets, and a bustle of people who seemed to be happier and better dressed. I suppose the public holiday mood also helped. That evening, Ilya, Alex Masur and I walked from the city down a long ramped cobbled roadway to the riverbank where we were joined by Ilya's wife Tatiana (Tanya) for a fine fish dinner on the water's edge. As dusk fell, we were serenaded by a nightingale.

Next morning, after a late breakfast we were joined by most of the original paediatric cardiac surgery team with the exception of Alex Masur who was on duty. After stopping at a grocery and liquor store for essential supplies we headed for a picnic in the country. This time our lunch included a generous supply of salads, cold pork, pickled fish, baked bread and some fruits. Clearly, the standard of living had improved a lot. That evening, I joined Tanya and her elder son, Kyrill, at the opera where we saw a production of *Onegin*. At the second interval we left the show and were joined by Ilya for an excellent dinner nearby.

At the Monday morning hospital assembly, which I dubbed the "prayer meeting", the director Knyshov gave one of his usual lengthy speeches and I later gave a little reply of my own, stressing my thanks for having been invited now and previously, the striking changes in the city, and my belief that such excellent teams of people were bound to do good work. We renewed acquaintanceship with three of the original Sydney team, that is Yemets, Masur, Perepeka, and his wife Irina, also a paediatric cardiologist.

After taking coffee with Academician Knyshov I scrubbed in with Ilya for a complex and difficult operation on a rare cardiac tumour, which he handled very well.

We spent an hour or two in an excellent art gallery situated in a former mansion of a pre-revolutionary industrialist, then drove to the luxurious dacha of another of Ilya's non-medical friends, a prosperous film director. Flushed by a lengthy session in the sauna the more enthusiastic guests dashed naked into the near freezing river for the traditional cool off.

Dinner began with first course of borscht with many toasts in vodka, followed by a walk to the river, then a second course of blinis and caviar with many more toasts and then a session of billiards accompanied by more Cognac. Fortunately, Tanya was the designated driver for the trip home.

Next morning, after assisting Ilya with a complex congenital case, we enjoyed a farewell department party with a big chocolate cake provided by the long-term scrub nurse Lyudmilla and Irina Perepeka, washed down by a bottle of brandy.

That evening Ilya and Tanya entertained Director Knyshov and his wife at the Yemets' apartment. After soup and salad, we had a walk around a rejuvenated convent nearby then ate a flattened chicken breast on a bed of vegetables – chicken Kyiv I suppose. Plenty of vodka, champagne and wine and many toasts. After dinner we were entertained by Ilya's 10-year-old son, Gleb, who played the piano very well with a preference for jazz and Gershwin, and then Ilya and his elder son Kyrill played some elegant violin duets. The following morning Ilya was tied up with final preparation for defence of his PhD thesis. I had the pleasure of being shown over a beautifully restored Orthodox church and a moving conducted tour through the nearby catacombs, containing the mummified bodies of hundreds of priests dating from around 1000 CE. Ilya joined me and his friend Danilo, in whose flat I was staying. Yet another church visit, then quick coffee and Cognac for lunch and there was just time for me to collect my bag and go to the airport. I stayed overnight in Zürich, was delayed in departure by a spectacular electrical storm, then flew via Riyadh to Abu Dhabi.

This brief 2001 visit to Kyiv was remarkable for the degree of recovery of the city since I had last been there, and for the excellent progress which the congenital heart team had made. They were still a somewhat uncomfortable part of the Cardiac Institute but their growing expertise and confidence were clearly evident.

2011 Kyiv visit

In 2011, long after I had retired from practice, I had a surprise phone call from Ilya, who announced that he had been appointed Minister for Health for Ukraine in addition to his duties as Director of a new Ukraine Children's Cardiac Centre. He had somehow secured and repaired an old pre-revolutionary tuberculosis hospital building. In addition to refurbishing the original three stories, he added two further floors above that, including an excellent operating room suite and intensive care area. Marilyn and I, along with Ilya's longstanding Strathfield supporter Christina Bilinsky and her partner Ian Goldsmith, were invited to visit, to celebrate 20 years of the paediatric cardiac work in Kyiv.

The new Children's Heart Institute was already performing over 1400 procedures per year, more than any similar centre in Europe. The standard of work was most impressive. Yemets had assembled a team of outstanding young cardiologists and surgeons provided with modern equipment and delivering an excellent service not only for Ukraine but also managing extensive referrals from nearby countries, mostly those of the former USSR. Operating rooms were small but functional, and the flow of surgery was efficient and effective. Nearby, a former army barracks had been transformed into a specialist hospital to serve a growing number of adult patients with congenital heart disease. This service was managed by Ilya's second-in-command and former trainee, Michael Bublik.

As usual, the social program was impressive and exhausting, including sightseeing in the now well rebuilt city with its spectacular gold domed churches. One evening there was a formal ceremony in a beautiful art gallery overlooking the river to celebrate the 20th anniversary of the Institute. An orchestra played, the medical bigwigs mingled with the great and good of Kyiv, and there was lots of champagne and many flowery speeches including those to thank me for my various small contributions as well as Christina Bylinski for her stalwart support, funding and supply of vital equipment in the early days.

Any spare moments in the evenings were filled with attendance at musical performances. One sunny weekend day all the available medical, surgical, technical and nursing staff held a big communal barbecue on the same river island I had visited 19 years earlier. While the boat man cooked up a monster fish stew consisting mostly of bones and potatoes, the young folk had fun with footballs, frisbees, even an air rifle for some target shooting. Everyone was in good appetite to deal with the roast meat and various salads.

Another day Ilya, Tatiana, Marilyn and I drove in Ilya's Mercedes 4WD out to another friend's fancy dacha by the river. Marilyn had a hard time because the other ladies present had no English, but I had an amusing day fishing from a speedboat, along with the hosts. The technique of fishing was a kind of jigging in which a small hook with a lure was lowered toward the bottom and reeled in using a rod. I never really got the hang of it, but the locals caught several small fish, which we later had for lunch. As the Dneiper River upstream still served as the cooling pond for the still-functioning Chernobyl reactors, we had fleeting concerns about radioactivity.

For our final long weekend, we flew with Tatiana to Crimea to stay at Ilya's so-called dacha at Foros. This fine newly built house, complete with sweeping staircase and grand piano, included sauna, swimming pool, elegant gardens, even a special stairway down to the chilly waters of the Black Sea where Ilya liked to cool off after his sauna.

Crimea was an excellent place to visit with few tourists but plenty to see. The Black Sea coastline here is of high, weathered rugged limestone cliffs, backed by the green Crimean mountains. Highlights included ancient Greek and Italian ruins, and some spectacular Orthodox churches perched on the mountains.

One guided sightseeing trip took us westward along the coast to Sevastopol and neighbouring Balaclava. Sevastopol is still the site of a major Soviet naval base, situated on a deep and capacious natural harbour. Even when, at the time of our visit, Crimea was part of Ukraine, the Russian military retained control of the city and it was a somewhat forbidding area. [All of Crimea was re-annexed to Russia in 2014].

Balaclava, headquarters of the British force during the Crimean War and rich in history, is a much smaller harbour but very attractive. One surprise was the opportunity to walk through a former Soviet submarine base situated in a long tunnel deep beneath the cliffs, a major Soviet naval asset with thick steel doors, supposedly making it safe against even nuclear weapons during the Cold War. Now it is a museum.

Another highlight was our stop on the ridge from which the English Generals overlooked and directed the calamitous charge of the Light Brigade. I always had a mental image of the "valley of death" as being a kind of canyon into which the ill-fated cavalry charged. In fact, it is a broad, open valley, now containing a few nondescript vineyards, wide open to the devastating artillery fire rained down on the assault from the surrounding hilltops. The engagement lasted a mere 20 minutes. A very moving and reflective experience for us.

We were joined for the rest of our stay by Ilya, who announced that he had resigned as Health Minister in frustration at being unable to execute his program of reforms.

We later returned to Balaclava where Ilya had engaged a fishing boat operated by a giant Russian and his boat boy. On a beautiful day we motored out of the harbour and along the coast for a short distance. Each of us was handed a rod and line, set up with about a dozen tiny unbaited hooks on a long leader. The idea was to let the heavy sinker take the leader to the bottom, then retrieve it with a jiggling motion which somehow attracted the sardines. It was not uncommon to hook half a dozen with one cast, so we soon had a plastic bucket nearly full of them. We anchored in the shelter of some of the weathered limestone pinnacles and enjoyed some Cognac while the boat boy gutted and fried the fresh morsels. The balance of the bottle completed our lunch. Delicious.

Next day, we drove east to Yalta, which had been a traditional Russian seaside resort since the days of Catherine the Great. In Soviet times it had many ugly waterfront sanatoria, which could be visited by the Russian workers, who were given a good holiday including enforced saunas, exercise and swimming, all regimented and supervised by the staff. Most of these sanatoria are now derelict but a few are being bought up by modern oligarchs and either rebuilt or transformed into very luxurious dachas.

We met up with the handsome Health Minister of Crimea [not the entire Ukraine] and his girlfriend, who joined us for a visit to the former Emperors' Livadia Palace, where we enjoyed a very generous lunch followed by a tour of the historic precinct. We sat at the table where Churchill, Roosevelt and Stalin determined how to carve up post-war Europe.

In a final grand gesture, Ilya invited us to the nearby winery of the last Czar. This was built on a suitable Imperial scale, with the great storage caverns excavated into the hillside, and its wide frontage embellished by an imposing limestone façade. The facility holds a million bottles, dating from 1876. We were treated to a tasting conducted by the director of the winery and his assistant. At the end, I was presented with a bottle of Crimean wine from the year of my birth, 1933. [A few years later we broached this bottle at my 80th birthday party, held at Alison's house at McMahon's Point. The ancient vintage was sound and sweet, and was, to my palate, a Tokay-like dessert wine.]

Yemets' return to Australia

In 2014, Ilya, his wife Tanya and son Gleb revisited Australia. After some time with their old sponsor Jack Olssen in Canberra they spent a few days to see the sights of Sydney. I accompanied Gleb and Ilya to the Westmead Children's Hospital where Ilya presented an interesting paper on his recent research into open heart surgery within a few hours of a baby's birth, using blood harvested from the umbilical cord to avoid use of donor blood. This talk was well-received.

At the weekend, Bruce Handmer kindly drove the Yemets family from their Macquarie Street hotel to Palm Beach. From there they took the ferry to Wagstaff, where Marilyn and I met them. They stayed a few nights with us at Killcare, where they greatly enjoyed the novelty of surfing.

A week at Hamilton Island in the Whitsundays completed their stay in Australia., something Ilya had anticipated for years.

Comment on Ilya Yemets

I taught about 70 advanced trainees in cardiac surgery. With very few exceptions, they have been highly successful, some of them outstandingly so. Ilya Yemets is one of a handful who stands out. He rose from an unusually difficult beginning and has achieved so much in a troubled and impoverished country, through his intelligence, drive, and incredible energy and creative talents.

Yemets was born in 1956 in the Vorkuta Gulag, a coalmining prison far from Moscow in Arctic Russia. He graduated in Medicine from Kyiv Medical University in 1979, later specialising in Cardiac Surgery in the Amosov Institute of Cardiac Surgery, Kyiv.

I have described his advanced training in paediatric cardiac surgery in several leading Western centres, including two stints with us in Sydney. He became chief of paediatric cardiac surgery at his old Institute in Kyiv.

In 2000 he was elected to the Ukrainian government and became Health Minister, but resigned in 2001 in frustration at his inability to carry out his required reforms in organisation of health services including administrative structures, training and certification.

By the time of my third visit in 2010, Ilya had established his own Children's Cardiac Centre, serving the whole of Ukrainc and accepting patients from surrounding countries.

In 2020, as the coronavirus epidemic began to sweep his country, he was co-opted as Health Minister, but again resigned, frustrated by his inability to appoint a preferred deputy.

At the time of writing, in mid-2020, Ilya Yemets was in his mid-60s, still energetic and creative, and may yet achieve even more in research and surgical practice. Despite his humble beginnings, he has been a marvellous pupil and a great teacher, organiser and leader.

[In February, 2023, it is distressing to record the ongoing invasion and destruction of Ukraine including its capital, Kiev. Yemets and his team continue to work in their Children's Cardiac Centre, sometimes under fire. An amazing man!]

Chapter 7: The Arabian Gulf

I have written the story of my semiretirement in the United Arab Emirate of Abu Dhabi in a separate book, "Arabian Days", largely compiled from my correspondence and journal entries.

Why did we go to this unfamiliar place? As I approached my mid-sixties I was on the lookout for a suitable job as a step-down towards full retirement. At the same time, I was becoming extremely frustrated by the administrative and political circumstances at the Children's Hospital and within the New South Wales Health organisation. Therefore, when I received an offer from Yousuph Nazer, an Indian colleague whom I had known from his days as a trainee at Prince Alfred, I considered it seriously.

After much negotiation and some procrastination, Marilyn and I flew to Abu Dhabi in January 1997 for an exploratory visit. The Emirate was alien but by no means unpleasant, an exotic culture in an inhospitable climate, with numerous challenges. Nevertheless, we both thought it would be a stimulating experience, within my capabilities. It presented a reasonable, if unconventional pathway to retirement. The Abu Dhabi Health Minister offered me a job as Head of Cardiac Surgery and Advisor to the Ministry and, after some lengthy haggling we agreed on conditions of employment. After spending most of 1997 extricating myself from Australian Hospital, University, and practice commitments, I began work in Abu Dhabi at the beginning of 1998.

The first half year was frustrating at many levels. After a month or so I was given reasonable temporary accommodation and Marilyn joined me. The process of negotiating for our permanent lodgings and preparing to move in to them took six months but finally we were ready to settle properly into our excellent apartment on the Corniche, fronting the waterfront of the Arabian Gulf.

As we settled our domestic arrangements, I was already comfortable in my Department at the Al Mafraq Hospital. Work was not very arduous as most of the operating was carried out by my colleagues, Dr Yousuph Nazer and Professor IM Rao. Each morning we made a formal round, then consulted with the physicians about potential patients, and spent any spare time in the operating room as spectators. There was usually some time for reading.

Over time I appreciated some of the pluses and minuses of the hospital. The physical facilities were fairly good as the hospital had been built to an Italian design only 15 years before. The equipment was a little out of date but adequate. Most of the staff had been recruited by Nazer and were competent and companionable. Nazer had trained in Trivandrum, later spent time at Royal Prince Alfred Hospital in Sydney and was an excellent coronary surgeon. Professor Rao, who had trained in Delhi and in Auckland and worked as a staff member in Portland, Oregon, was expert at all forms of paediatric cardiac surgery. The staff doctors who functioned as registrars were mainly Indians. One interesting character was a Somali doctor, Italian educated and Moscow trained. We had a Syrian resident doctor on our team who was mostly useful as an Arabic interpreter.

Our scrub nurses were Egyptian, Iranian and Mauritian and the perfusionists were Iranian and Indians. Ward nurses were mainly Filipinas.

The Cardiologists were an interesting group. The senior ones were Iranian and Indian, including two that I had known from visiting Vellore many years earlier. Our main Paediatric Cardiology colleague was a highly competent Keralese Indian. They were good to work with, with the exception of one Emirati who lacked some insight and the necessary collegial attributes. All in all, a competent and enjoyable team.

The Administration setup was understandably foreign to me. The Hospital Director was a well-connected local man, somewhat impetuous and autocratic, but intelligent and mostly good-humoured. He was directly responsible to the Ministry, which was located in the city. The Health Minister, an Iranian, was also personal physician to the country's Ruler. Because the Ruler was himself ageing and increasingly unwell, both of them spent long periods seeking medical attention abroad. The Minister therefore was often distracted, inaccessible, and not available for day-to-day management.

The lesser administrative staff in the ministry building were a source of great frustration. Many of the senior ones were Egyptian and usually unhelpful and often obstructively antagonistic. A little further down the chain were some Filipino and Indian clerks who were not necessarily unfriendly but lacked authority to be of much help.

In my book on the subject, I have described at some length the cultural and religious features of the Emirates. During my time, at the turn-of-the-century, it was a fascinating society, mediaeval in structure, deeply religious, authoritarian, defensive, and sometimes threatening. On the other hand, 30 years of exploitation of the oil fields had made it about the richest country on earth in per capita terms, with interesting architecture and rapidly developing infrastructure, and offering a feeling of personal security beyond my expectations.

Once settled in, Marilyn and I enjoyed nearly four years there. The work itself was challenging and very satisfying, as cardiac surgery always is. Hours were not onerous and I was usually home for a late lunch by about three o'clock, leaving time for a siesta during the hottest part of the afternoon. We maintained a reasonable level of fitness, mostly based on swimming at a local hotel pool during summer and walking during thc winter evenings.

There was plenty of time for reading. Several local restaurants provided variety in the form of Italian, Indian, Lebanese, Chinese and International cuisine, in addition to our simple home-cooked meals made with excellent, readily available ingredients from most parts of the world.

We managed two visits back to Australia each year and used most of our time during each trip on catching up with family, business commitments, and usually a professional conference.

A highlight of our time in the Gulf was to have family members and friends visit. Marilyn's sister Roslyn and my sister Rosemary came twice each, as did John and Alison and their families. We also had brief visits from John and Charlotte Overton, Brian Morgan, and Richard Hawker. Depending on the time available we turned these visits into opportunities to tour the Emirates and the neighbouring country of Oman so that in the end we had seen much of the Arabian Peninsula.

My original contract was for two years and I extended that for one additional year. By then it was becoming clear that there was little more to achieve in surgery, and we were beginning to miss our children and grandchildren. With some difficulty I got my Hospital Director to agree that I should retire towards the end of 2001.

Negotiating the bureaucratic nightmare of separation from my contract was as tedious as settling in had been in the first place. The 9/11 terrorist raid on the Twin Towers in New York was very upsetting within the multi-ethnic community of the Gulf. We were relieved and happy to be home before the end of 2001.

Tim in 1998

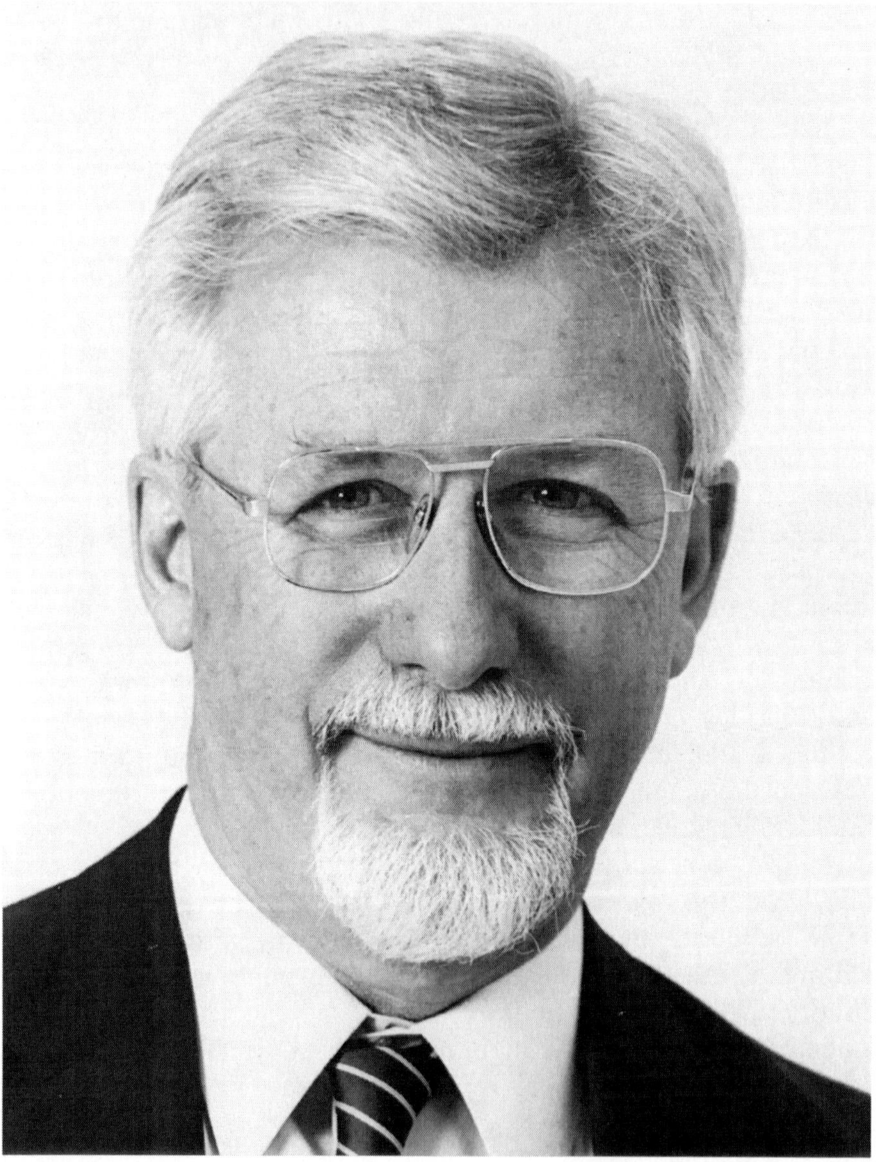

Chapter 8: Retirement years

"The undesirable outcomes of ageing vary from person to person, but, on average, elderly individuals experience significant losses in both physical and mental functioning. Yet they don't let the declines undermine their happiness. In fact – and here's the paradox – old age produces the opposite result: the elderly feel happier than they did when younger, stronger, and healthier... When it comes to dealing with all the negativity in their lives, seniors have decided that they just don't have time for it, literally. They've come to desire a time of emotional contentment for the remaining years and they take deliberative steps to achieve it... The elderly go more frequently and fully to the locations inside and outside themselves populated by mood lifting personal experiences. To a greater extent than younger individuals, seniors recall positive memories, entertain pleasant thoughts, seek out and retain favourable information, search for and gaze at happy faces, and focus on the upsides of their consumer products": Robert Cialdini: Pre-suasion: a revolutionary way to influence and persuade.

Amen: I never intended to continue working beyond the proper time. Our adventure in the Middle East had been intended as a step towards full retirement, and it was successful. By the year 2001, at the age of 68 years, I thought I had achieved as much as I was likely to achieve in Abu Dhabi. I was physically weary, and no longer enjoying the stress of operative surgery as much. The political frustrations and anxieties of that time and place were also beginning to take their toll.

Having arrived back in Australia at the end of that year we took some time to settle back in our home, and into a slower routine. The house itself needed painting and various other maintenance. I needed to buy a car, and we enjoyed re-establishing contact with our families. My recollection is of a relief of tension, and a growing appreciation of the pleasures of everyday existence.

I reaffirmed a previous conviction that there is a time and place for each of us to retire. Individuals must decide that time for themselves. For high-pressure occupations such as heart surgery which demands qualities such as dexterity, persistence, and intellectual sharpness, nobody should hang on for too long. Individuals vary a lot and it is difficult to generalise. Certainly a few surgeons continue to do good work into their 70s but others should have quit earlier. We all hope that our friends or anaesthetists will "tap us on the shoulder" in good time but, in the end, each of us is responsible for their own decision.

Consultancies

Consultancy is one of the small perks of retirement. A letter or phone call arrives requesting or pleading for help in some thorny problem, not necessarily directly related to one's former workplace, but usually touching on supposed professional or management expertise.

Brisbane

Shortly after I returned from Abu Dhabi, I received a call from a friend of Bev Clarke's who asked if I would join his small group to review some planning by Theiss, the large construction group, for Wesley Private Hospital in Brisbane. The original Wesley Hospital building was quite elegantly designed, but like many hospitals, had made additions piecemeal and opportunistically when needs were pressing or when funds became available. The resulting campus had become fairly confused and our task was part of an overall attempt to rationalise the present assets and future development plans. We were briefed by management, interviewed many key players in administration and various services, and tried to propose useful future solutions. This arm's length thinking is enjoyable and potentially valuable in solving larger-order problems unrelated to the day-to-day task.

By chance, several years later, I was engaged by the same hospital to give an independent assessment of an apparent cluster of post-operative infections in the Cardiac Surgery department. Infection after clean cardiac surgery should be unusual, ideally zero, but some cases inevitably occur. They do not come at regular intervals so there is always a chance of three or four in an apparent cluster. That may indicate a significant systemic failure of preventive measures. The possibility that the infection control procedures are not fully effective is unsettling, frightening and disruptive and may result in overt or covert finger-pointing and sapping of morale.

I spent two or three days reviewing the individual cases and sat in on the operations, all of which were carried out with the usual proper safeguards. I interviewed the infection control officer, the central sterilising department staff, and as many of the key support people as I could. In brief, I could not identify a specific problem. No single surgeon accounted for all of the cases. Happily, the complications did not continue or recur so if there was a systems failure it must have resolved before I arrived and without my help. Such an outcome may have been intellectually frustrating, but it was practically reassuring.

Another Brisbane consultancy was of a different scale. I was co-opted by Craig Mellis, a former colleague from the Children's Hospital at Camperdown. Craig was a Paediatric Chest Physician who had returned to university, gained a PhD in Epidemiology and subsequently became Dean of the new Medical School at Bond University on the Gold Coast.

Mellis had been called in to recommend a solution to a perceived problem with Paediatric Cardiology and Cardiac Surgery services in Brisbane and the whole of Queensland. There were some long-standing grievances and ill feeling between the Cardiac Surgeons who were based at Prince Charles Hospital, the major public cardiac centre, the Intensivists who had been seconded from Brisbane Children's Hospital, and various other players. Without suggesting individual blame, it became clear that physical arrangements were not ideal, many of the personalities were in conflict, communications were not robust and healthy, and something had to give.

Our consultancy team included Mellis, myself, and the distinguished Melbourne Paediatric Intensivist, Frank Shann, among others. We took several days to visit the various institutions and consult as widely as possible. Given the personalities, loyalties, traditions, regional tensions, geographical arrangements in Brisbane, and the usual high emotional content of paediatric matters, this was the kind of problem in which the fresh outlook of an outside team might be helpful.

In coming to our recommendations, we were influenced by our knowledge of long-standing arrangements in Sydney and Melbourne. As Paediatricians

we did not favour having Paediatric services performed at specialist adult hospitals, which had been the prevailing arrangement in Brisbane. Further, we were
of one mind that it was far better to concentrate such a highly specialised paediatric service in one centralised position, as in Melbourne. We sought to avoid at all costs the Balkanisation that had developed for historic and personality reasons in Sydney, where resources had been divided between one larger and one lesser Service, to the persisting detriment of both.

In principle we advised the Queensland government that a new Paediatric Cardiac Service should be established at a single site, with outreach medical services in regional centres and outlying areas of the city. We were not in a position to recommend any particular location, nor did we recommend any individual staff members who might be recruited.

No single site fulfilled every requirement and the Queensland Government in its wisdom chose to establish a new department at the Mater Children's Hospital in South Brisbane. At the time of writing (2015) a new purpose-built Children's Hospital is being erected on that campus. The existing Brisbane paediatric cardiac surgeons chose not to participate, and Graham Nunn, my long-standing colleague in Sydney, was recruited to head the new Department.

For their new service the Mater Hospital wished to recruit another surgeon, and their choice was a young American, Dr Tom Karl. At this time, regulations required that Karl needed to hold the Fellowship of the Royal Australasian College of Surgeons. This should have been a formality, as he was an experienced surgeon, having held positions in Melbourne and several major Children's Hospitals in the United States, but his election to Fellowship was conditional on subsequent formal performance evaluations. For this purpose, I was appointed by the College of Surgeons to make regular site visits over two years.

Mater Hospital Management also asked me to evaluate their new cardiac surgery program on behalf of the Hospital and Queensland Health. For a while I became a regular visitor to Brisbane, staying overnight and flying home via Newcastle the next day.

Before each visit I was sent complete clinical details of all operations and of all significant complications and deaths. Caseload rapidly rose to a satisfactory level, results were well within accepted international norms, and Tom Karl settled well into the Brisbane scene. On each visit I would review each adverse outcome with the staff and interview all key team members. I also sat in on surgery to observe Dr Karl in action. My regular reports were accepted both by the College of Surgeons and by the Queensland health authorities.

What I learned

Although sometimes derided as a temporising way of palming off sticky management decisions, consultancies of these sorts can be very useful. Outsiders should offer a fresh perspective on a difficult problem, they can circumvent personality clashes, and ideally they can propose effective potential solutions.

To be asked to serve on such committees is a privilege. The intellectual challenge is different from the daily problem-solving of medical practice. It requires a generalised, abstract, arm's-length and dispassionate intellectual approach, informed by experience and an open mind.

Teaching in retirement: Institute of Clinical Excellence

I had not long settled in after returning from Abu Dhabi when I had a call from Ian O'Rourke, a former General Surgery colleague at Westmead Hospital in the 1980s. He had taken up a position as head of the Institute for Clinical Excellence (ICE), recently established by New South Wales Health, and was charged with implementing a program of Root Cause Analysis which was to be applied to all major clinical errors in New South Wales hospitals.

During the closing years of the 20th Century there had been increasing awareness of the problem of potentially preventable mistakes in the medical system, specifically in hospitals. It had become clear that many deaths and complications were not matters of chance so much as human, equipment, or system failures. The traditional reflexive medical denial of error had given way to a more realistic acceptance that in Medicine, as in all human endeavours, error is frequent, inevitable to a degree, codifiable and potentially preventable or manageable.

Root Cause Analysis is an engineering technique used to investigate failures. It was among the measures used to study aviation accidents and more recently had been applied successfully to investigate adverse events in the US Veterans Administration Hospital system, a program implemented by the charming and persuasive former astronaut, Jim Bagian.

Accidents in Medicine, as in engineering and elsewhere, are generally the result of a chain of errors arising from one or often more root causes, which can be identified and addressed. Recognising that errors commonly arise from recurring causes, the VA mandated that both the investigations and the proposed solutions were made compulsory throughout their nationwide system. The program had been highly effective.

The NSW Health's Institute for Clinical Excellence (ICE) team was due to teach one of its first sessions at Bathurst Hospital on the coming weekend. I was asked to fill in at short notice for Tom Hugh. I became part of the team and remained so for about three years.

Operating from NSW Health offices at North Sydney, Michael O'Rourke as Head of ICE, was joined by Nurse Educator Sarah Michael and Paul Douglas, a medical doctor from John Hunter Hospital in Newcastle, both of whom had made pilgrimage to the US to absorb the Message and translate it to an Australian idiom. Retired General Surgeon Tom Hugh, Anaesthetist John Overton, and a former Director of Nursing, Jan Stow, were joined by me as part time teachers in a program to be rolled out over several years.

Each training session lasted a day and a half and combined various set pieces and workshops which had been adapted from the American program. Over two or three years we preached our message at most of the major city hospitals and regional centres, including in Long Bay Prison. The early sessions were a learning experience for our faculty as well as the trainees, but we steadily improved.

The system we were to implement ran along these lines:

Any adverse clinical event was to be reported within the hospital. A committee selected from Administration, Nursing, Medicine, and any other relevant discipline was given a standard set of procedures to be followed. The event was to be classified and, if judged to be significant by dint of severity or likelihood of recurrence, would be further studied. A timeline would be agreed to, defining what had actually happened and when. Then, working backwards from the outcome, a series of chains of causal events would be established, and a small number of significant "root causes" identified.

Proposed solutions and preventative measures could then be devised and implemented.

Our teaching was generally well received, especially in rural and regional areas. The procedures were not unduly complicated but demanded an open mind. They were not universally grasped or welcome; a few individuals in some hospitals were inflexible or overtly hostile.

As in the United States, our system was supposed to be compulsory, but I was never completely convinced that the results had been effectively promulgated and fully enforced. Thus we may not have achieved quite as much as we had hoped.

Eventually, the New South Wales Health ICE program was subsumed by a more ambitious Commonwealth of Australia scheme called the Clinical Excellence Commission (CEC). Michael O'Rourke had recently died and was replaced by the very able retired surgeon, Cliff Hughes. It was a bigger, more expensive, more comprehensive, hopefully more effective program and John Overton and I were no longer required as teachers.

Anatomy

Anatomy teaching began with a phone call from George Ramsay-Stewart. George is an old General Surgery colleague from Royal Prince Alfred Hospital from whom I had not heard for about 30 years. "Good day, Tim, how have you been?… Look, I am starting this course in Anatomy by Whole Body Dissection, and I need your help".

Teaching of Anatomy to undergraduate students, more specifically the lack of it, had been an increasingly sore point among surgeons for many years. By about 1980 medical schools around Australia and in much of the world were struggling with their curricula. Many medical courses had been reduced in length from six years to five. At the same time, advances in medical knowledge and basic science presented more and more material that deserved to be incorporated in the Medicine curriculum. As part of the perceived solution, anatomical dissection had been almost completely abandoned in most medical schools.

The contention was that "in our day" many hundreds of hours had been allotted to dissection of the body, often with limited direction, and usually with little lasting recall of the details. It was argued that the relevant bits of anatomy could be taught or absorbed along with other basic sciences in the course of the "problem based learning" which was the pedagogic fashion of the day. So this major subject matter, about which many do not need to know much, was not being taught well to anybody at all, including those who in their future career would need to know a great deal of it, especially Surgeons, Anaesthetists and Imaging specialists, among others. Surgeons were especially scathing of this turn of events, but as someone said about the weather "Everybody bitches about it but nobody does anything about it".

Ramsay-Stewart was the one who actually did do something and, through his force of argument and personality, had reinstated an Option course in Anatomy by Dissection, offered to incoming final year medical students at Sydney University. George's difficulty was in finding teachers who had time to spare and who also knew sufficient Anatomy to impart it to others. Hence his recruitment of several retired surgeons.

When I first knew George as a Registrar and later a Junior Surgeon, he was a bustling, ginger haired enthusiast. In retirement, now greyed, but still rubicund and rotund, his enthusiasm had not waned, and he pursued his goals with energy and forceful persistence. He had been appointed Professor of Surgical Anatomy and allotted a small room as an office in the Anatomy Department. This contained a desk, a phone, a computer, a tea tray, and not much else, certainly not a personal assistant.

The lofty dissecting rooms in the historic sandstone Anderson-Stewart "Old Medical School" building had been brutally partitioned into pokey tutorial rooms but George restored and refurbished them and added modern overhead-mounted computer screens to display the textbook diagrams. Unfortunately, at that stage, the major dissecting room did not have proper air-conditioning apart from a kind of jerry-rigged arrangement connected by ducting to the half open windows. In January afternoons this contraption produced plenty of noise but did not extract much heat.

The first courses got underway about the end of 2008. In the beginning there were about 30 students, plus half a dozen Demonstrators recruited from advanced trainees in surgery, and a handful of us senior Supervisors. The course ran in December and was repeated in January. The courses were well received, with the students nearly all showing enthusiasm and talent. This was not surprising, given that they were bright people anyway, and were self-selected for this course. George ran a tight ship, beginning each day with a presentation by one of the students of the work to be done that day. Several hours of dissection followed. After a brief lunch break we convened for a lecture on some topic, often by one of the senior Supervisors, and then worked well into the afternoon. For my part, I found it physically and intellectually tiring but exhilarating.

Over time, the course evolved and simplified. The two courses per summer were condensed to a single course in January. Many of the Supervisors dropped out after a year or two. Some categories, especially general surgeons, had been overrepresented, and probably felt they had little to contribute. The core specialist groups such as neurosurgeons, orthopaedic surgeons, and cardiothoracic surgeons continued faithfully but over the years began to dwindle through illness and death. The number of students was also trimmed and we were able to fit into one of the smaller dissecting rooms which was well air-conditioned and more comfortable.

One bonus was my renewed association with David Johnson, my old colleague at the Children's Hospital and Westmead Hospital. Often we both attended, but, if one or the other was otherwise committed we could relieve one another.

The textbook we were using, *Cunningham's Manual of Practical Anatomy*, first published in 1883, was quite impractical for heart anatomy, probably reflecting the ancient lineage of this traditional textbook. With the concurrence and support of Johnson and George Ramsay-Stewart, I rewrote a short section of the book to describe a much more practical and up-to-date approach to dissection of the heart. The new material was typed out and distributed so it could be used to guide the study. This was a success, and in 2015 I made minor improvements to the text.

For several years we taught pro bono, and the University generously allowed us to park free of charge in the grounds. Eventually, George secured an agreement with the Department of Anatomy to pay all the Supervisors, collectively, the equivalent of a single Lecturer's salary. In practice, I got one tenth of a salary, which was fair. The only downside was the bureaucracy required in signing up as an employee, paying superannuation, and accounting for the transactions for tax purposes. After functioning satisfactorily for about two years this arrangement was terminated by the University as part of an economy drive and we were dismissed from paid employment with a nice thank you letter. I had been considering retirement anyway, but I still believe in the cause of proper anatomy teaching. David Johnson took over, with the agreement that I could cover for him if he were not available.

A few months later my son John had the bright idea that I might use the new facilities at Macquarie University Medical School to make a video to demonstrate my revised heart dissection. John then asked me to spend a couple of days each year as one of the Supervisors for the new Macquarie Medical Sciences Diploma in Anatomy course. That was enjoyable so I accepted an appointment as Adjunct Professor and have taught further courses.

What did I learn?

I enjoy teaching. It is more relaxed in retirement and the instructor can take time to convey their enthusiasm for the subject. The calibre of present medical and surgical students is impressive; they are receptive and enthusiastic and often demonstrative in their thanks.

Travel highlights

As Marilyn and I approached retirement we began to dream of spending significant time and resources seeing as much as possible of Australia and other parts of the world. Some of our most memorable experiences are described in Appendix 3: Travel. Here is a sampler:

Mungo Lakes, 2005

To attend a College of Surgeons conference we had planned to take our Subaru Forester on the train to Perth and drive home. Unfortunately, the car was too high to be taken by train on the Sydney to Adelaide leg, so we decided to drive across the Hay Plains. Our second overnight stop was at Balranald. By chance I saw a flyer on the bedroom door advertising Mungo Lakes National Park so we decided to divert through there the following day. It is about a hundred kilometres off the main highway and the roads are rough and dusty. The "lake" is a former anabranch or diversion of the Murrumbidgee River, dry for millennia. These ancient lakes are characterised by flat bottoms and rimmed on the northern and eastern sides by ancient sand dunes, formed by then prevailing winds.

The Park entrance is near the old sheep station buildings and contains some simple introductory posters. The nearby semi-derelict shearing shed is interesting in itself. There are also some self-service cabins available but no other amenities. The main points of interest are accessed by driving across the old lakebed for a couple of miles to reach the ancient dunes, the site of Aboriginal camps thought to be at least 30,000 years old. Successive erosion of the old dune structure reveals middens and old fire pits, sufficiently well preserved to give an excellent sense of some of the old campsites and their inhabitants enjoying feasts of the fish caught back in the days when the lakes held water. This was the site of discovery of the skeleton of Mungo woman, later followed by other skeletal remains of a people perhaps antedating the current Aboriginal race. It is a spiritual place, remote, simple and moving. Unfortunately, the flies were so numerous and aggressive that lunch was limited to a small tin of cold baked beans each, shovelled in quickly to thwart most of the dipterous competition.

Langgi Beach, Kimberley Coast, 2014

We were greeted on Langgi Beach by the local mob of Aborigines. Their main spokesman was tall, eloquent and persuasive. They would have liked to sell some of their paintings. These were well executed but the prices, up to $1500, seemed a bit steep. I think they sold one or two. At low tide we were able to enter, one by one, an extraordinary cave, richly embellished by wall paintings including "contact art", probably depicting Dutch visitors.

At low tide this was a remarkable and beautiful area of broad sand beaches, red bluffs, deep green foliage, the gorge with little creeks entering it, and a striking group of eroded sandstone columns, said by the Aborigines to be their ancestors, including the chief and his wife and a battlefield. Assuming this yarn was true, the battle had left plenty of dead!

As we left, our hosts staged a smoking ceremony for our benefit. A little fire was set, then lit by the maître d' using his BIK cigarette lighter. Some green acacia leaves were added to provide the smoke, through which we dutifully filed to receive the good wishes of the elders and a daub of ochre on the forehead.

Japan, 2005

After we arrived half a day late because of a delayed flight, the fast train to Tokyo and a connecting commuter train transferred us to our hotel at Kawasaki. Next morning, after a traditional Japanese breakfast of miso, fish, etc, we headed downtown for an extensive walk to find our land legs and get attuned to the go-go rhythm of Japan. In a park we bumped into a TV film crew shooting a children's gardening show, then found some fellows drumming in the park. A couple of derelicts lay asleep by the pathway, one with his socks drying on a nearby shrub.

Finland, 2007

Finland was perhaps the most distinctive of the Baltic countries. Outside the main cities it is still thinly populated, with agriculture and forestry predominating. Dominated by Russia throughout most of the 19th and early 20th centuries, it still has a slightly Russian feel to it, with lakeside dachas and their saunas, timber or stone churches which look Orthodox but are often Lutheran, and a somewhat taciturn people.

After we had enjoyed the modern city of Helsinki and its more traditional surrounds, our trip took us partly by waterways but mostly by train northward to the Arctic Circle. Santa Claus village was a disappointing tourist trap, but I did not really expect to meet the bearded old fraud in person. One memorable highlight was an outdoors zoo. A very personable young guide showed us around. At first it was a let-down because the nocturnal animals could not be seen and the birds were confined to a smallish aviary, but the big animals, especially the polar bears, brown bears and reindeer were excellent and the lynx really spectacular.

Isle of Man, 2012

We had seen the flyer for IOM Trikes in our hotel lobby, and our guide, Owen, organised for us to be picked up by them at Peel. We were not dressed for the occasion but our host kitted us out in strong waxed textile black coats, and helmets fitted with intercom. We were seated side-by-side behind our driver, whose seat was that of a conventional motorcycle with long chopper style front forks. With a 1200 cc car engine there was more than enough power, but we toddled along sedately without exceeding 80kph. [The Tourist Trophy has been run annually since 1909, with some nine years missed due to the two World Wars. Modern riders complete the 60km course at average speeds well above 200kph, reaching 300kph on the straight, hard to believe when the race is run on ordinary narrow roads through village streets.] There were plenty of stops along the way for us to see points of interest and to be told stories of the big bike race. A Boy's Own Adventure for me!

Wales, 2012

Much of our time in Wales was cool and drizzly, but that did not prevent our enjoyment of numerous scenic trips on old-narrow gauge tramways, often of only about two feet [60 cm] gauge, and generally drawn by small historic steam locomotives.

Until recently this area of Wales was the world centre of slate mining. We saw plenty of the old pits, as well as the workshops in which the rocks were cleaved into individual slates for transport all over the world. The industry has more recently been undercut by the Chinese substitute. On one of the slate tours, I noted as we climbed into the forest in increasing rain that it was a slate grey day with slate grey rain amid slate grey clouds beside waste slate roads with houses whose roofs, walls, and floors were all built of slate.

Isle of Skye, Isles of Lewis and Harris, 2012

The Isle of Skye is romantic territory for those of us with Scottish blood, who grew up with the legends of Bonnie Prince Charlie. It is a ruggedly beautiful place with black-faced sheep and some long-horned Highland cattle, the dramatic Cuillin mountains, and rugged multicoloured "tartan" cliffs.

A couple of days later we took the ferry across the Minch to the Isle of Harris. I enjoyed watching a display of hand-loom weaving, which they still used to manufacture the beautiful Harris Tweed suitings. An afternoon bus trip took us North through the bleak countryside to the evocative town of Stornoway. This is an ancient and strategic port with substantial quayside buildings.

Next day we visited Callaway, interesting for its stone circles and old Fort building, and for the village of refurbished black houses in various states of repair. These are the low walled solid stone houses with a thatch secured by cables weighted down by huge stones to retain the roof during the winter gales. We looked through one of the black houses. One end was reserved for the cow byre, while a primitive little kitchen had a small smoky peat fire smouldering on a simple central hearth on the floor beneath an opening in the roof for the smoke. Curtained sleeping quarters were at the opposite end from the cows.

Staffa, 2012

On the island of Staffa spectacular basalt formations form flutes in various orientations, including a Giant's Causeway, and a narrow walk around the base of the cliff to Fingal's Cave. This was an enthralling grotto with its deep clear water, blue jellyfish, a high fluted vault, and amazing echoes. Very cold!

Cultural activities in retirement

One of the best things about retirement is its abundant time for non-work activities, especially cultural activities.

Reading and writing

I have always been a voracious reader. These days free time and the cornucopia of Amazon provide a bottomless supply of material and opportunity. Since newspapers have become available online it is not even necessary to go out to buy the daily edition. The challenge is to find sufficient discipline not to fritter away time on repetitive blogs and similar trash.

Fiction is a pleasant diversion, but technical and educational material helps keep the mind open to fresh ideas and points of view. My son John and I often swap ideas about books and papers, although I admit that he now contributes the lion's share of new ideas.

A vague ambition to write a Memoir took a long time to advance beyond a few unfocussed jottings.

In 2009, on a whim, I joined one of Helen Menzies' Life Writing classes. This was an interesting experience in itself as a group of older people, mostly women, were chivvied through the process of turning memories into written words. Helen is a talented teacher who uses enthusiasm, energy, and a sympathetic manner to introduce the tricks of getting started and putting something on the page. Each session lasted a couple of hours with a half-time coffee break, and included warmup sessions which Helen calls sprints, some short exercises on given topics, and some longer periods of writing from real life experiences. The disciplined experience of committing some stories to paper, reading them back for critique among the class members, and editing and expanding the material for homework between classes was effective. At the end of the course we held a session of readings for our families and friends, with rewards of polite applause, with food and drink to follow.

About five years later I re-joined one of Helen's classes for a tune-up. As before, she was an adept teacher. If anything, the class members were even more capable, perhaps that much younger and less inhibited.

Encouraged by the writing classes, I took up the task of collating and editing my papers from our period in Abu Dhabi. By combining daily diaries, journal entries, and letters to family and friends, along with some newly written bridging material, I finally completed a hefty book, "Arabian Days". This was received courteously by my family members and one or two friends.

Music and Theatre

During our working life Marilyn and I attended concerts, ballets and plays, subscribing from time to time to seasons of them. We came late to opera but enjoy it very much. The difficulty was always finding time and energy. To finish work and rush to the theatre in time for a quick drink, dinner and show was always problematic. I have slept through more Second Acts than most people.

In retirement there is plenty of time, so the only real limitations are getting to the city to enjoy the show, and the expense of tickets and accommodation where necessary. A spur of the moment decision to go to an opera or musical show in the city often necessitates an overnight stay. Local productions, both amateur and professional, have often been enjoyable. One of the most consistent treats has been the baroque music of the Brandenburg Orchestra, originally suggested to us by John. For me, this is about the most accessible music of all and the combination of an excellent group of musicians, mostly playing period instruments, in the beautiful Sydney Recital Hall, has been a source of endless enjoyment and satisfaction. We have subscribed to about five concerts a year for many years now and will continue to do so as long as possible.

Cinema did not really hold my attention until recent years. Now that we have time we go to the movies, usually at Avoca but sometimes at Ettalong, and enjoy our selective choices.

U3A

University of the Third Age is a valuable organisation which enlists retired academics and other enthusiastic teachers who are prepared to present their subjects to all who choose to come, at a nominal cost. The offerings vary in quality, seriousness, and competence but there is usually something of interest and worth attending. Courses run from single-day sessions through to a dozen or more lectures at intervals of a week or two. We have enjoyed many different topics including travel, history, technology, and literature. Highlights for me were several series of highly professional lectures on Philosophy presented by Georg Illi; informative and a great stimulus to further reading.

For a few years I presented one-day sessions on various topics of interest, with the collaboration of my son, John. Our lectures were often broadly related to Safety, which is one of John's special areas of expertise. We tried to make the shows entertaining, avoiding talking-head presentations or traditional didactic lectures in favour of interactive and stimulating stuff. These were well received and popular, so it was with some regret that I had to give them up after I suffered strokes, coinciding with John's opening of his new Macquarie University Hospital. Collaboration with my son was a big part of the pleasure.

Family and friends

I am by nature a loner, often comfortable with my own company and thoughts. But then, I have had the luxury of a supportive family in most of my endeavours. Beyond immediate family, many of my friendships developed and prospered at work; indeed the fostering and maintenance of productive associations is the key to a lot of professional success. Outside of work, my range of friends is not very large but I value them deeply.

I have described earlier the immediate and extended family in which I grew up as a child. Both my mother and father were excellent parents, loving and supportive, instilling positive values and behaviour, using discipline in a limited and effective way, and inculcating valued social qualities. Our aunts and uncles were always there as we grew up and I can only wonder at their forbearance. They were older than my parents, unmarried themselves and must have found us trying at times.

My brother and two sisters and I have always been on good terms, although we are separated in age by a span of a dozen years. Hence we have been friendly, but perhaps not as close as some siblings. Each of us went off to boarding school at around the age of 11 or 12 and that also shaped our relationships – it is one of the rarely articulated consequences of leaving home for school, especially for country raised children.

At the time of writing, Poppy is 93 years of age and has in the past few years suffered some significant illnesses. She has survived in reasonable health and in good spirits, and with her intellect intact. After living alone, in the Queensland mining town of Moura where she worked for much of her adult life as a teacher, she now lives in a retirement village in nearby Biloela, where she is often visited. by some loyal friends and neighbours. We enjoy chatting by phone, but only see one another face-to-face every few years.

Sadly, my younger brother Gaine died recently at the age of is 84, after a full life on the farm where we grew up. He represented his community as Mayor in local government, pursued business interests including a sawmill, and enjoyed close ties with his wife, Ruth, and sons Bill and Bob. We miss him.

Rosemary is the youngest, and lives alone in her excellent retirement village at nearby Davistown. She is as independent and strong willed as ever.

We make new friends at school, mostly dictated by common interests. My three or four closest mates there were "scholars"; although we took part in sports we were not particularly talented or interested in them. Hurlstone did not have a very strong alumni network, and I lost touch quickly with all of them except for Barry Wren, my fellow medical undergraduate at Sydney University. Even there, Barry and I were not very close because he lived at Wesley College while I went to St Andrew's.

University friends were mostly College friends. Sadly, of my closest associates, most died early. John Kennaway was killed in a car accident, as was Jim Cox. Bill Bevan committed suicide a few years later. I remain on good terms with others, like Lindsay Roberts and Ian Pryde, but we see each other very infrequently. Life got busier, work got harder, family commitments developed.

Marilyn and I were married at a young age and within three years had our two children. It has been a great source of pride and satisfaction to see our children develop, to remain close to them as we age, in more recent years to share with them their own adulthood and developing families, and to remain good friends with them and with all the grandchildren.

John applied himself diligently to gain entry to Medical School, even repeating final year of school. Since then his career has gone from strength to strength. Having graduated from Sydney University, qualifying MBBS, BSc (Med), MSc (Med) he completed surgical training in Australia before spending a few years in USA perfecting the emerging skills of laparoscopic surgery while specialising in Colorectal Surgery. En passant he worked for six months with Johnson & Johnson research engineers in Cincinnati. As well as a successful and busy practice in Colorectal Surgery, he has cultivated an interest in safety and accident prevention in surgery, and also technical innovations in surgery. He has a well-deserved reputation as an outstanding lateral thinker, with his skill in applying concepts from altogether different disciplines to medical problems. This was doubtless one of the reasons for his being recruited for the team which created the new Private Hospital and Medical Clinic at Macquarie University in Sydney. Here he had a major role in the conceptual and physical planning of the new institutions as well as staff recruitment and becoming Head of Surgery. He has more recently been promoted to Associate Dean of Clinical Medicine in Macquarie University.

Alison has taken the less technical route, graduating BA Dip Ed at Sydney University and acquiring numerous further qualifications, mostly concentrating on communication, education and learning. She qualified from a graduate *Sydney Morning Herald* Cadetship to work as a journalist with Fairfax Corporation. As well as raising a very talented family and teaching for a short while, she has combined her educational and journalistic skills in public relations at Sydney University, Australian Catholic University and Wenona, an independent day and board school for girls. She worked as a contractor with Justice NSW, then as Director of Media and Communications with International Grammar School in Sydney. She writes fiction in her sparse spare time.

Our five healthy, delightful and intelligent grandchildren are a blessing, and we admire and support them all. They certainly cover a range of talents:

Casey with his BSc (Honours First Class and University Medal) from the University of Sydney and his PhD from Caltech, his formidable intellect and idiosyncratic view of the world, recently resigned from NASA in Los Angeles to found Terraform Industries, a startup which aims to mine carbon from the atmosphere. With his wife, Dr Christine Corbett Moran, he enjoys parenting our great grandson, Yosemite and great granddaughter, Sequoia.

Marcus, MBBS (Honours First Class, University Medal, UWS), applies his reliably solid competence to his work as a Urologist and Head of Department in Newcastle, where he and his wife Charlotte are raising their children, George and Edward.

Annie with her multitalented expressiveness, BA in Philosophy (Honours First Class), at the University of Sydney, has completed her PhD in the History and Philosophy of Science at the University of Sydney. She is well connected in the global space industry and is working with the NSW Department of Premier and Cabinet.

Tom has a BA majoring in Psychology from the University of Sydney and a Graduate Diploma of Psychology and Master of Clinical Psychology from Deakin University. He is currently practising Clinical Psychology while tackling a challenging PhD project with the University of Melbourne.

Hannah has completed a BA in Psychology and Sociology at the University of Melbourne and a Doctor of Physiotherapy at Macquarie University, is hard at work in Physiotherapy.

Those grandchildren are all serious students and practitioners. Not a loser among them!

Most of my friends are former colleagues; hardly surprising when so much of one's waking hours are spent at work. John Overton and I spent so long working together, mutually supportive both professionally and politically, day and night, through thick and thin, that it is not surprising that his is one of the relationships most dear to me. David Baines is a younger anaesthetist with whom I continue to be friends, a good man to have on your side in a scrap, and a solid citizen. Overton, Baines and I meet together a few times a year, mostly for lunch and usually with a few other anaesthetic and surgical retirees or near retirees. Paediatric Cardiologist Gary Sholler is another of the younger colleagues with whom I occasionally still talk or meet for coffee or a meal – our relationship is more one of professional and administrative fellowship.

Of my few non-professional friends over the years, sadly most have long gone. For many decades there was simply no time for socialising outside of work.

One interesting group with whom I still meet most months is a lunch club called the Sydney Birthday Club. Nearly a dozen years ago I was invited to join by Ray Hyslop, an Obstetrics and Gynaecology acquaintance from our time in training at Royal Prince Alfred Hospital. John Overton is another member. The strength of this club is that it includes senior people, mostly retired, from such diverse fields as Aviation, Medicine, Law, Banking and Commerce, Military, and professional musicians and academics.

In summary, I enjoy a handful of close friendships, I delight in my family, and I can be happy alone or with my wife. It may not be fashionable but it suits us.

Ageing and infirmity

"Old age isn't so bad when you consider the alternative."
—Maurice Chevalier

Luck deals the cards. Life expectancy is largely determined by inheritance, then misfortunes, accidents and injuries will come to bear. Although my parents did not live very long lives, most of their siblings did.

To some degree we can and should manage the risks. Diet and exercise help reduce preventable illness and control weight. Vaccinations prevent or attenuate many infections. Exercise helps maintain mobility and reduces injuries. General medical care by a trusted General Practitioner can detect and modify risk factors such as hypertension, hypercholesterolaemia and impending organ failure. My preference is to use these services in a calibrated way, being realistic in one's expectations, conscientious in following suggestions and treatments, but keeping medical care in perspective. It is part of the means to a healthy ageing, not an end in itself.

I lean toward Stoicism, accepting the inevitability of some changes associated with ageing, while utilising all sensible means of mitigating them. Visual acuity diminishes, at first slowly but then more rapidly with the onset of cataracts. Upgrading of spectacles, maintenance of good lighting, and regular check-ups make a huge difference to quality-of-life. Cataract surgery is one of the true miracles of our times. I experienced slow deterioration of hearing, presbycusis, over a long time. Preservation of communication and simple enjoyment of one's surroundings are worth the effort and inconvenience of hearing aids: they are helpful, though not as miraculous as spectacles.

Some other fading faculties such as agility and balance have no specific treatment but can be compensated to some extent by prudent anticipation, exercise and household aids such as shower rails and handgrips.

Memory loss is interesting. In my case it seems more a matter of slowing of recall than total loss of memories. I suppose this is the earliest manifestation, and things may get worse over time.

My main experience of serious illness was a series of strokes over several months in 2009. The third of these was sufficiently serious to require hospitalisation and has left me with significant residual disability. The right upper limb is worst affected, especially right hand movements. This is frustrating because it affects my handwriting and fine motor control in general. Dictation software helps somewhat in overcoming this difficulty but is not always convenient and can be hilariously inaccurate.

After it became clear that the cause of my strokes was intermittent atrial fibrillation [a rapid irregular heart rhythm], I was invited to participate in an international collaborative trial of one of the experimental new oral anticoagulants, Edoxaban. This was a rewarding experience. For over three years, each month I attended my Neurologist's rooms where a dedicated and highly competent practice nurse made the necessary observations and collected specimens. At the end of the study period, during which this particular drug was shown to be effective in prolonging life and avoiding the quaintly named "adverse events", I changed to the already approved new oral anticoagulant, dabigatran, and have taken it ever since. There must be a significant amount of luck involved, but this new class of drugs is a major advance in medical treatment. They are easy to take, require no regular attendance for blood tests and have proven effective in preventing recurrence of stroke.

What I learned

Enjoy life and health while you can. Bless the good fortune, take credit where it is due, accept professional and personal help with respect and gratitude, and do not waste time grieving over what might have been.

Philosophical musings

"Know thyself"

Although I was confident that it was a quote from the Bible, this injunction or variants of it have been expressed by thinkers since Thales of Miletas. One of my motives. for writing this memoir has been to try to crystallise the "meaning of it all".

I have no religious conviction whatever and feel comfortably confident that there is no afterlife to anticipate or be concerned about. To that extent, I have no fear of death, which is just as well, given that it is inevitable and unavoidable and not too far away.

That is not to minimise a well-informed apprehension about the possible process of dying. Quickly and without too much suffering would be nice, but we do not get to choose. Prolonged incapacity is the thing to be dreaded. Some progressive mental deterioration seems inevitable with ageing but dementia of the degree that seriously changes one's identity and social capacity is of concern. Closely related to this is the effect on one's family, friends and carers.

Physical incapacity is also a progressive and cumulative inevitability which can be adapted to in part. Realistic acceptance of what is possible is the key. At some point increasing physical dependence on the care of others might preclude a worthwhile existence.

Marilyn and I have made whatever reasonable formal provisions we can for these eventualities. Last Wills and Testaments, Advance Directives and similar documents have been drawn up, signed and witnessed and are held by our Solicitor. One small surprise as we worked through this formality was the practical impossibility of specifying all or many of the various conditions in which decisions might have to be made, and hence the impossibility of writing "dos and don'ts" for those who might have the unpleasant task of making those decisions. There are simply too many permutations of options for them to be specified in advance, so the directives must be broadly expressed.

It is reassuring to have discussed this matter more than once with my son John. He certainly has the intellectual and professional capacity to act appropriately when and if called to do so, and I fully trust his judgement. That is not to minimise or diminish the responsibility which may be his.

Closure of life cycle

Contemplating life's end brings a curious calmness independent of any thought of an afterlife. Stoic thinkers have always known this; it is merely an expression of its inevitability.

It is certainly a time for reflective assessment of the life lived. Achievements and failures, good times and bad, challenges and responses, satisfactions and regrets, trials and imperfections.

As the marvellous journey nears its end it is time to acknowledge indebtedness to parents and all other family members, teachers and mentors and many other supporters, friends and a few foes, wins and losses. I hope that I have done my best with the hand I was dealt and would not change much of it even if I could.

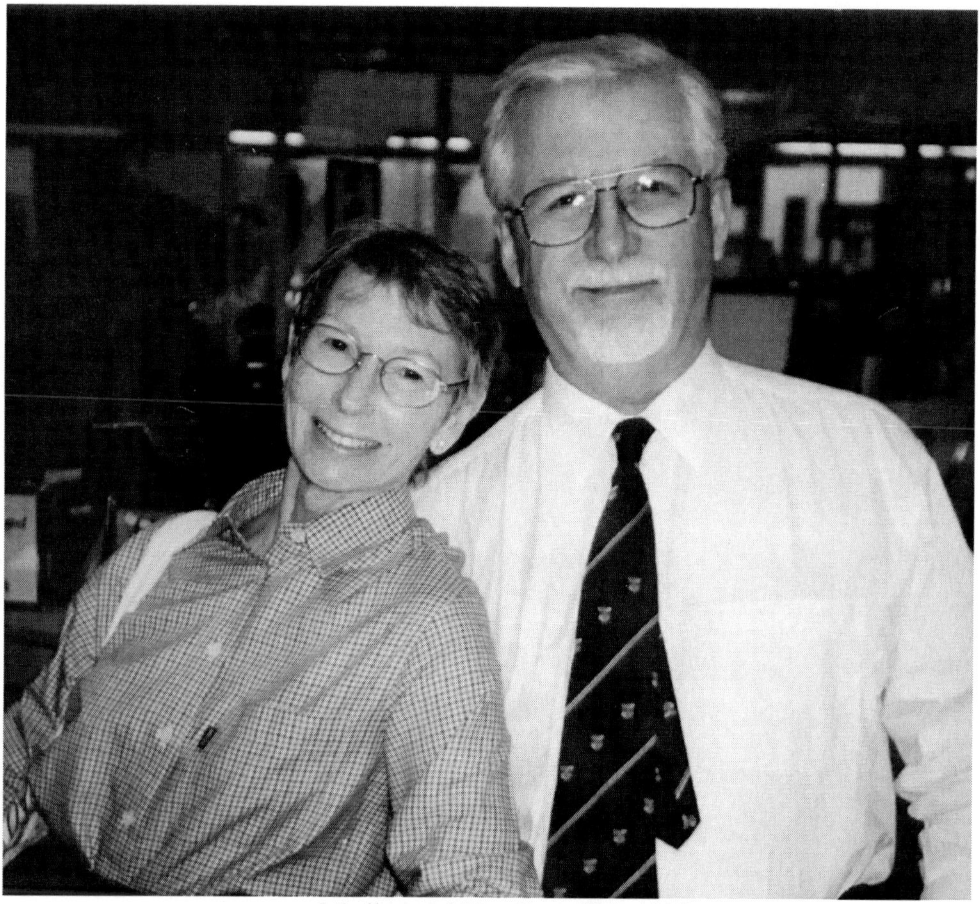

Marilyn and Tim Cartmill in 1998

Introduction to Appendices

Many of my life experiences do not fit well into the chronological structure of this memoir. In some cases, the content is medical or technical and may not appeal to all readers. Additionally, many of the themes are general or philosophical or extend over long periods of time, and do not belong in any particular time period. For these reasons I have assembled this collection of appendices covering some diverse topics which I hope may be of interest.

Appendix 1: Cardiac surgery

A brief history of cardiac surgery

There was a certain inevitability about the development of open heart surgery in the 1950s.

Since ancient times the heart had been considered off-limits for surgery. A very few heart wounds had been sutured successfully but even touching the heart was likely to cause ventricular fibrillation and death. In 1935, Sir Henry Souttar in London performed mitral valvotomy, using his index finger to dilate the valve which had been scarred and narrowed by Rheumatic Fever. Subsequent attempts failed because neither diagnosis nor surgery nor anaesthesia were sufficiently developed to support this feat before World War II. Near the end of the war Dwight Harken successfully removed foreign bodies from the hearts of more than one hundred US servicemen, without loss of any patient. By then intermittent positive pressure ventilation with anaesthesia had been perfected allowing respiration to be maintained during open chest surgery, antibiotics were available, and lung surgery was rapidly developing.

Almost simultaneously in 1948, Russell Brock in London, Charles Bailey in Philadelphia, and Dwight Harken in Boston repeated the mitral valve operation with success. Specialised knives and dilators were developed to facilitate "blind" valvotomy procedures guided by a finger introduced through the left atrial appendage.

At Johns Hopkins Hospital in Baltimore, Alfred Blalock developed his palliative shunt "Blue Baby" operation to increase pulmonary blood flow for cyanotic congenital heart disease, especially tetralogy of Fallot. Blalock's operation, previously described under "1967", diverted blood from a subclavian artery, which normally would supply an arm, into the pulmonary artery, so increasing the blood flow to the lungs. The Blalock shunt was effective in alleviating symptoms but did not "cure" the abnormality.

True open-heart surgery began with simple procedures, such as repair of atrial septal defect, using inflow occlusion [temporary obstruction of the superior and inferior venae cavae, the great veins which drain blood into the heart] to achieve circulatory arrest under total body hypothermia. Bill Bigelow in Toronto, Henry Swan in Denver and Clarence Crafoord in Stockholm lowered body temperature to 30 to 32 degrees C by cooling the surface of the body. This permitted the circulation to be interrupted, allowing the heart to empty and be opened for a brief period. Impressive though this was, it allowed only four to eight minutes in which to perform the intracardiac part of the repair, ruling out all but the simplest procedures.

What was required was a suite of techniques allowing a longer period of complete arrest of the heart. For this an apparatus was needed to maintain the patient's circulation and gas exchange of oxygen and carbon dioxide for prolonged periods, bypassing heart and lungs: a "Heart-lung machine" or Pump-Oxygenator. Basic principles of maintaining perfusion and oxygenation of individual organs had been devised and used for bench-top physiology experiments many years before; the challenge was to scale up the equipment and render it fit for safe clinical use.

By the 1950s most of the necessary technologies became available. Blood banking was reliable. Heparin prevented blood from clotting and was reversible. This application was essential to prevent blood from clotting in the apparatus. Plastics were used for tubing and other components of the heart-lung machine. Practical pumps included the sigma motor pump, normally used in industries such as wineries, which utilised cam-driven "fingers" to milk fluids along a tube, and a scaled up development of DeBakey's roller pump, originally devised for direct blood transfusion from a donor to a patient.

The first successful open-heart operations using extracorporeal circulation and cardiopulmonary bypass were the cross-circulation procedures of Walt Lillehei in Minneapolis. One parent was used as a donor to supply oxygenated blood for whole-body perfusion of an infant or child. Some wags pointed out that these were the first operations with a possible mortality rate of 200%. Ethical concern about using live donor perfusion promoted development of various artificial oxygenators, of which the most successful of that era were the bubble oxygenator developed in Minneapolis by deWall, the rotating disc oxygenator developed by Kay and Cross, and a vertical screen oxygenator devised by Gibbon in Philadelphia and further refined by Kirklin at the Mayo Clinic with the collaboration of the IBM corporation.

It was now possible to perform deliberate surgery within the non-functioning, bypassed heart without the critical time limits and risks of total body hypothermia and circulatory arrest. The limitations of these techniques took some time to determine, and much of the knowledge about pathology, instrumentation, materials, and surgical techniques was still to be developed.

Beginning of open heart surgery at Royal Prince Alfred Hospital

In early 1957 I assisted Frank Mills who was conducting experiments in the animal laboratory in the Sydney University New Medical School to prepare for open heart surgery using cardiopulmonary bypass. The technical staff had secured a sigma motor pump and set up a Lillehei-deWall bubble oxygenator circuit. This apparatus was constructed of lengths of plastic tubing of various dimensions, supported by retort stands and other standard lab equipment. Briefly, the idea was to drain venous blood from the animal into a large vertical chamber where it was mixed with oxygen, causing foaming and gas exchange. This froth rose and spilled over into an obliquely inclined length of tubing into which a silicone solution had been sprayed to reduce surface tension and break the bubbles. The now mostly liquid blood was allowed to settle through a spiral helix which also acted as a reservoir. The oxygenated blood, hopefully now free of residual bubbles, was pumped back to the arterial side of the animal's circulation. In Minneapolis and elsewhere this circuit had by then been used for about two years for open heart surgery in humans.

By 1956, Sir Edward Hallstrom, philanthropist and supporter of the Hallstrom Institute of Cardiology at Royal Prince Alfred Hospital, had undertaken to sponsor a team of American surgeons to introduce the open-heart techniques in Sydney (delayed until 1957). Hallstrom also provided funds to purchase the necessary equipment.

Cardiothoracic surgery had reached an interesting stage of development at Prince Alfred. The general surgeon John McMahon managed most of the lung surgery. An enclosed veranda of his Ward D1 had been equipped as a

Thoracic Unit. Fred Neische also performed some chest operations, mainly oesophago-gastric surgery.

Frank Mills had pioneered closed mitral valvotomy in Australia, and later performed palliative shunt operations for tetralogy of Fallot (Blalock's "Blue Baby" operations). As the mitral caseload grew, Harley [Mick] Turnbull and Paul Tomlinson were recruited to perform this operation. By 1957 Turnbull had retired from the field. Sandy Grant had recently returned to Sydney following postgraduate training in thoracic surgery in London, and was assisting McMahon and Mills, as well as beginning to establish his own practice. Notably, he had completed a successful series of repairs of coarctation, or narrowing, of the aorta, which did not require a pump-oxygenator.

The Page Chest Pavilion was opened towards the end of 1956, and the New Zealander, Rowan Nicks, was recruited as its first Staff Surgeon. So, as the open-heart surgery era dawned at Royal Prince Alfred Hospital, four of the existing surgeons had a legitimate interest in it. McMahon and Neische had done no cardiac surgery, but Mills, Grant, Tomlinson, and Nicks were vitally concerned.

I have previously described (under "Royal Prince Alfred Hospital" above) how I came to be involved with the open-heart surgery program in 1957, first assisting Frank Mills in preparatory work in the dog lab of the New Medical School. Our experimental subjects were failed racing greyhounds. They were generally docile to handle although we were careful to use muzzles. Anaesthesia was induced with Pentobarbital, a long endotracheal tube was introduced, and ventilation maintained with a simple respirator. The femoral artery was exposed, heparin injected to prevent clotting, and the heart-lung machine connected to the arterial circulation. The heart was exposed through a chest incision. Plastic cannulae were inserted in the superior and inferior vena cava and connected to the venous side of the artificial circulation. If all went well, the -various tubing connections could be unclamped and the pump started. That sounds simple, and it is now performed thousands of times every day throughout the world, but we all had to learn the disciplines involved in opening the clamps, starting the pumps, beginning and completing cardiac bypass, stopping the pumps, re-clamping the tubing, and removing the cannulae, before administering protamine to reverse the action of the heparin and allow the blood to clot. There were many potential pitfalls in these techniques, including the maintenance of the circulation, avoidance of air bubbles and embolization and protection of the organs involved.

Gaining familiarity with this complex new technology was not easy. The apparatus was conceptually simple but unsophisticated, with absolutely no failsafe controls. It was all too easy in the excitement of the moment for someone to start the pump while the tubing was still clamped, resulting in a spectacular explosion of arterial blood which sprayed over most of the laboratory and the operators. Similarly disastrous was failure to maintain the occlusion of the tubing until the correct moment, draining all blood from the subject: a messy business but part of the necessary technical and mental preparation. Slowly we made progress and gained some practical familiarity with the technique. With hindsight, we should have done much more of this kind of preparatory drill.

While Mills and I were practising those most basic techniques, Rowan Nicks had undertaken a lengthy study tour of leading departments including those in London, Stockholm and North America. He visited Russell Brock, Clarence Crafoord, Bill Bigelow, John Kirklin, Michael DeBakey and Denton Cooley, Henry Swan, and Frank Gerbode. This was an excellent selection of the leading players in the field at that time. Rowan's conscientious but barely legible notebooks of this tour are held in the archives at Royal Prince Alfred Hospital.

As described above, I was to be the Surgical Registrar covering the American surgeons' visit at the end of 1957, and Louis Bernstein would be my medical (Cardiological) counterpart. When the big crates of equipment arrived we opened them with interest but had insufficient knowledge to assemble or use the contents. Most impressive was the Electronics for Medicine monitor console, a 6-foot-high instrument rack containing the amplifiers and displays. Two 6-inch orange oscilloscopes occupied the top panels. One of these was exclusively used for "balancing the galvanometers", a black art requiring the adjustment of a couple of knobs to create as perfect a Lissajous figure-of-eight as possible on the screen. The other scope, utilising a beam splitter, continuously and simultaneously displayed an electrocardiogram, an arterial, and a venous pressure trace.

The heart-lung machine was a "Mark" brand Vertical Screen Pump-Oxygenator. A square trolley was set low to the floor to provide an adequate syphon to drain the venous lines. An eye-level shelf held voltage transformers, AC-DC rectifiers, and controls for the pumps. Two simple DeBakey pumps, one to maintain flow in the oxygenator and one for arterial inflow, were driven by DC motors. The oxygenator was a simplified vertical screen design similar in principle to the Mayo Clinic's, but without the automated controls. Blood was pumped to a diffuser at the top of an array of stainless steel mesh screens suspended within a Perspex box where it was exposed to a humidified oxygen and carbon dioxide mixture. Establishing the capillary films of blood on the screens required practice. The oxygenator was completely filled with saline. At a shouted command this saline was rapidly drained into a bucket by means of a wide-bore plastic tube colloquially known as the "elephant's trunk". Simultaneously, blood was pumped to the top of the screens. If all went well the blood would course down the screens in a nice continuous layer as long as the recirculating pump kept running. A fine stainless steel mesh in a Perspex chamber served as a simple arterial line filter. The venous reservoir was also made of Perspex, and a separate cardiotomy reservoir received blood scavenged from a left-heart vent and hand-held suckers from the operative field, allowing it to settle before being reintroduced into the circuit. All in all, a dramatic piece of equipment.

"Hi, Ah'm Henry Bahnsen", announced that tall, gaunt, broadly grinning American as he strode forward to shake my hand. That was my first meeting with Hank, the senior of the two Americans who had come from Johns Hopkins Hospital in Baltimore to help us set up the open heart surgery program at Prince Alfred in 1957. Bahnsen and Frank Spencer had started open heart surgery in Dr Alfred Blalock's Department of Surgery at Johns Hopkins Hospital in Baltimore, Maryland. Bahnsen and Spencer were about 37 and 33 years of age at that time.

Both surgeons threw themselves into the task of preparing the heart-lung machine and the special monitoring equipment and demonstrating their use in the animal laboratory. None of us had seen such enthusiasm and intensity before. They had planned four animal experiments to bed in the techniques in preparation for the human operations.

It is not easy to perform operations of this magnitude on experimental animals, and (in hindsight) it is not surprising that the first three animals did not survive. Our team members were somewhat dejected and the usual doomsayers within the hospital were delighted. Bahnsen and Spencer remained confident and decided that the fourth animal would simply be put on cardiopulmonary bypass without any operation within the heart, restored to normal circulation and allowed to recover. This experiment went smoothly and the animal survived uneventfully. It was reasonable to proceed.

Before undertaking the heart-lung machine operations in the hospital, it had been decided to demonstrate the hypothermia/inflow occlusion technique described above to close simple atrial septal defects. In this method, no artificial circulation is used. Body temperature is reduced to about 30C, the heart is exposed, the great veins (superior and inferior vena cava) are temporarily obstructed allowing the heart to empty. This affords up to about eight minutes in which to open the atrium, suture the defect and close the heart. It is a reproducible system but requires speed, decisiveness, and dexterity.

Our first inflow occlusion patient was anaesthetised and placed in a one-man rubber dinghy on top of the operating table so that he could be covered in ice and water to reduce the body temperature. The ice and meltwater were drained and the dinghy deflated to allow the operation to proceed. All went well and Bahnsen repaired the atrial septal defect within the required time. The patient's temperature had drifted a little lower than the target of 30C. The heart did not immediately recover on refilling but developed ventricular fibrillation. This abnormal rhythm causes the ventricles of the heart to quiver in an uncoordinated way instead of their usual rhythmic contraction and relaxation. No blood is pumped, and this problem is fatal if not reversed.

An electrical defibrillator had been purchased to manage this possible complication. This apparatus, only recently developed, was a bulky instrument powered by the 240V AC supply. Simple electronic controls allowed AC shocks of selected duration and voltage be applied to the heart via metal paddles. [It does not seem to be widely understood that the present direct current (DC) defibrillator was introduced several years after 1957. It delivered a much shorter shock at a higher voltage, using less energy and causing much less damage to the heart and other body tissues.]

While circulation was maintained by "cardiac massage", compressing it by hand to simulate contraction, the paddles were hastily connected and applied to the heart and a brief shock given. Fibrillation stopped, but recurred immediately.

This was serious. Bahnsen, and, after he had tired, his assistants, continued to compress the ventricles rhythmically to maintain an artificial circulation. In an attempt to raise the patient's temperature, the rubber dinghy was re-inflated and filled with hot water to warm the body while warm normal saline was poured over the heart. Repeated efforts to achieve defibrillation led to the same result; evident brief defibrillation followed by immediate recurrence of the problem. As the period of attempted resuscitation spread beyond an hour the observers grew more and more despondent. Many got dressed and crept away, but Bahnsen refused to give up. Others of the surgeons scrubbed in to relieve him in continuing cardiac massage.

After about one and a half hours Spencer suggested a desperate measure of which he had heard or read. In extreme emergency such as this it might be worth connecting the defibrillator paddles directly to the AC mains power socket, and simply switching the power on and off rapidly at the wall. Cardiology technician George Latham quickly connected the cables. By then the operating team members and their clothing were saturated with spilled saline, creating a serious risk of electrocution. One surgeon held one paddle, Bahnsen held the other and everyone else stood clear. At Bahnsen's order the switch was thrown. The anaesthetist, Bruce Clifton, who had been steadying the metal Waters' canister anaesthetic apparatus in his bare hands, cried out and was thrown back against the wall. "Turn it off!" Bahnsen shouted. The heart was beating normally! No one was seriously injured. The patient recovered with no apparent ill effects and has only recently died of old age. A triumph of courage, persistence, and ingenuity over adversity.

Frank Mills, Frank Spencer and George Latham later deduced that the defibrillator was continuing to deliver a trickle of electrical current leakage after the intentional brief high-voltage shock had been given to the heart. This was considered to be a defect in that particular device. Latham was able to correct the problem and the surgeons demonstrated in the animal laboratory that the defibrillator was now safe and effective.

Four patients in all had atrial septal defects repaired using hypothermia and inflow occlusion, while eight open heart operations were performed using the heart-lung machine. All of the patients were children or young adults with fairly simple heart defects. All twelve patients survived, a fine result for those days, indeed better than our American surgeons had achieved back home. My main role in all this was to care for the patients in the post-operative period, along with Bernstein. Maybe it was an example of the blind leading the blind, but success bred success.

Hank Bahnson later became Head of Surgery at Pittsburgh, and we were fortunate to have him back in Sydney to celebrate the 25th anniversary of our early triumphs. Frank Spencer became Head of Surgery at Cornell University in New York and made many contributions to cardiac surgery, particularly coronary artery surgery. What a taste of the American Way!

Implantable cardiac pacemakers

One of my early minor interests was the developing field of artificial cardiac pacemakers.

A 70-year-old retired electrical engineer called Eric Miller developed Stokes-Adams attacks. Adams and Stokes, two Dublin doctors in the first half of the 19th century, described the syndrome of loss of consciousness accompanied by a very slow pulse rate. Miller hoped that his fainting could be relieved by electrical stimulation of his heart.

We already had some experience of electrical heart pacing. When open-heart surgery began in Minneapolis in 1954, an occasional patient suffered heart block due to injury to the conduction tissue, called the bundle of His, which transmits the electrical cardiac impulse from the atrium to the ventricle. It is not the flow of blood which is "blocked", but the actual electrical signal which transmits a pulse from the atrium to the ventricle to cause the two chambers to work in sequence at the appropriate rate.

Fortunately, this surgical heart block is often only temporary, so if the heart is kept beating for a few hours or days the patient can recover. In Minneapolis they connected an ordinary laboratory electrical pulse generator to the heart with a braided stainless steel surgical suture. That was effective, and soon simple pulse generators for clinical use became available, at first housed in a big box and powered from the wall socket but soon refined to a six-by-four inch size and powered by ordinary dry batteries. These early pacemakers worked satisfactorily for a few hours but were unreliable for longer periods. The batteries soon went flat, the circuits were potentially hazardous, and the simple steel wires soon broke. Enter Miller's friend, Keith Jeffcoat.

Jeffcoat was one of a group of interesting people who had worked at Woomera rocket range, developing tracking and telemetry equipment. I knew of him as a contributor to *Radio and Hobbies* magazine. He had been working with the Children's Hospital in Sydney to improve their electronic monitors and pacemakers.

One of my tasks was to develop an animal model of heart block. I thought it would be easy to damage the atrioventricular conducting His bundle of a normal dog, but it proved quite difficult. This is odd, because it is all too easy to cause heart block when you are operating on the inside of an abnormal human heart: dead easy. Eventually we provided some animals and Jeffcoat and his colleagues refined the electrodes so that they would not break, and also to optimise the impedance, (a measure of opposition to AC current flow), of the leads and the means of connection to the heart.

For the electrode system Jeffcoat used a single steel helix wrapped around a nylon core, similar to the copper wire cords used in the telephone handsets of the day. This was a success; the electrodes were now predictable in their performance and worked reliably for years at a time.

My old boss, Rowan Nicks, operated to place one of these new electrodes on Eric Miller's heart, leading it out through the skin of the chest and connecting it to one of Jeffcoat's pacemakers. Miller was very pleased with the result. He got Jeffcoat to arrange a big external switch so that, even through thick winter clothing, he could turn it on for himself when he felt a bit funny when driving his car. At night he had to rely on his wife to switch the device on when needed. Miller and Jeffcoat reasoned that if you already had an electrical device directly connected with the heart via a wire it should be possible to monitor the electrocardiograph and set up circuitry which would turn the pacemaker on and off automatically when it was needed.

Nicks reported this case in the *Medical Journal of Australia* in 1962. Almost as an afterthought he included a paragraph mentioning the idea that it should be possible to automate this "pacemaker on demand" function. Many years later this was the subject of a huge legal patent case in USA.

Another tinkerer in the field of pacemaking was the American engineer Wilson Greatbatch. He made a fully implantable pacemaker in about 1962. From then on successful implantable models were made and used in the USA, Sweden, and the UK. They were simple pulse generators powered by mercury cells, set to a fixed rate of about 70 beats per minute, often competing with the patient's own heartbeats and potentially causing dangerous abnormal rhythms. Much work remained to be done.

Jeffcoat suggested the pacemaker project as a suitable line of research and development for a new Australian company, Telectronics (a contraction of Television and Electronics). Their stated ambition was "to develop, design, manufacture, sell and service electronic measuring, controlling and recording equipment for science and industry". Not a bad mission statement! Noel Gray was Managing Director and chief financier, and the self-taught engineer Geoff Wickham was Technical Director.

Their first batch of implantable pacemakers was made in 1965. They were powered by four Mallory mercury cells and contained a circuit board with a couple of transistors and a few other components, the whole thing encapsulated in a moulded acrylic package. Three of these pacemakers were implanted in patients and worked for between three weeks and eight months.

After further refinement the pacemaker became more reliable but still about the size of a pack of cards and quite heavy. It was implanted under the skin much as is done today, usually in the little depression under the clavicle. At first the connecting wire was sewn to the outside of the heart, but we soon learned how to introduce the electrode through a vein and follow it on x-ray fluoroscopy to advance it into the interior of the apex of the right ventricle. One early refinement was to incorporate a magnetic reed switch so at follow-up we could use a horseshoe magnet to adjust the width of the electrical signal remotely to either half or one millisecond to determine the minimum effective signal.

In 1967 Telectronics became part of Paul Trainor's company, Nucleus. Trainor provided financial, entrepreneurial and management resources to allow the company to grow and to adequately fund research and development.

In the years 1967 to '69 Geoff Wickham and his team solved several big problems. The mercury batteries had never been satisfactory. Over long periods, electrolyte leakage caused shorting of individual cells and sometimes damage to other circuit components. Geoff's first solution was to hermetically seal the battery pack to isolate it from the other components. Even then, water vapour from the patient's body tissues could penetrate through the epoxy resin capsule, sometimes causing the batteries to swell, burst their casing and cause ghastly inflammation of the surrounding tissues. To solve this fluid ingress, engineer David Cowdery developed a titanium casing to enclose the whole pacemaker unit, along with an ingenious means to argon arc weld the metal shell without damaging the circuitry. Geoff and I reported this work in 1971.

We learned that AWA was developing a facility in South Australia to make integrated circuits. Wickham, with David Money of AWA, designed a special integrated circuit pacemaker chip, printing most of the electronic components on the one chip, simplifying manufacture, hugely improving reliability, and saving power.

About this time Wilson Greatbatch, mentioned above, adapted the lithium iodide battery to pacemaking, and Telectronics soon incorporated this advance.

Our little Australian company at Lane Cove had within a few years introduced four major elements of modern pacemakers:

- The demand pacing concept
- External adjustment
- Titanium encapsulation to prevent fluid ingress
- Integrated circuits.

These inventions, plus the lithium iodide battery, were incorporated in the model 120 which appeared in 1974 and set the standard for all future pacemakers. One of this model worked for 17 years. Pacemakers were soon miniaturised to about the size of two 50-cent pieces side-by-side, quite light, occupying little space, and connected to the heart by long lasting reliable electrode wires.

From 1974 to 1978 Telectronics acquired subsidiaries in US, Canada, France, Great Britain, and Argentina for manufacture, sales and distribution and had become the second-largest pacemaker manufacturer in the world.

To quote from Geoff Wickham's memoir: "By 1978 ... the basic technology of cardiac pacemaking was mature, comprising microelectronic circuitry and hermetic sealing of the electronics and battery in a titanium case to provide a narrow 0.5 millisecond stimulating impulse to the heart. These … characteristics were innovations from Telectronics".

Cardiac transplantation

Often, when I meet a new acquaintance, one of their first questions is: "did you do any cardiac transplants?" My honest answer is "not many". But here is the story of my brief but intense interest in the topic.

The idea of organ transplantation was "in the wind" in the 1960s. Kidney transplantation had become widely established, with successful and well-regulated programs established in Australia.

Cardiac transplantation was a greater challenge because, unlike a kidney, the transplanted heart would need to recover full function by the end of the operation, and there was a very short interval of time in which the donor heart might be recovered and implanted. [Patients with kidney failure could be managed successfully almost indefinitely by dialysis techniques but long-term artificial circulation had not been attempted at that time. Above all, criteria for declaration of death of the donor also had not been established.]

It was a sensation when Christian Barnard successfully transplanted a heart for Louis Washkanski in Cape Town in December 1967. Although the patient died 19 days later of complications of immunosuppression, the precedent triggered worldwide activity.

After Barnard's case Norman Shumway at Stanford began human transplants. Barnard operated a second case, while many other surgeons were quick to follow.

At Royal Prince Alfred Hospital in Sydney we decided to study what had been achieved overseas and to establish a team to build proficiency in the technique and to learn how to deal with medical aspect s of patient care.

With the support of Prof John Lowenthal, then President of the Cardiac Society of Australia, cardiologist Louis Bernstein, anaesthetist Brian Clarke and I were supported to travel to several overseas centres to assess the situation. In 1968 we three flew to Cape Town via Perth, Mauritius and Johannesburg and visited the Groote Schure Hospital. Chris Barnard and his brother Marius kindly shared their knowledge and showed us their highly professional operation suite. We visited the animal laboratory in which baboons were being used to investigate production of anti-lymphocytic globulin for possible use as an immunosuppression agent to combat organ rejection. We also met and talked with Barnard's second cardiac transplant recipient who was making a good recovery at that stage.

In London we received the usual friendly reception from Donald Ross at the National Heart Hospital. In Houston we visited both Denton Cooley and Mike DeBakey. In New York at Maimonides Hospital. we had the pleasure of meeting Adrian Kantrowitz. Kantrowitz had performed the first cardiac transplant on an infant but unfortunately it was not successful.

At Stanford, California, we met Norman Shumway and his excellent team. Shumway, along with a former colleague Richard Lower, had been experimenting with cardiac transplants in animals for many years. He had already refined his topical hypothermia method of preserving the heart without blood supply for an hour or more [immersing the heart in frozen saline slush to cool it and reduce the need for oxygen and nutrients] with good recovery. Barnard had relied heavily on this work but Shumway had not proceeded with human transplants because the ethical question of how to determine the time of death had not been established. [Over time, brain death became accepted as a defining criterion of time of death, rather than lack of heartbeat, which had held for time immemorial.]

Bernstein, Clarke and I returned to Sydney, reported our findings, and stated our opinions. It was reasonable to set up a team, begin laboratory work, and prepare to incorporate transplantation into clinical practice. We recruited a small and excellent group of nurses, and worked out technical details of the operation using pigs, which were available to us at that time. As expected, the surgery was not unduly demanding, but preparing for overall patient management, as well as the logistics of donor management and transportation, was quite daunting. By this time cardiac transplantation was enjoying a worldwide wave of "irrational exuberance" with at least 100 cases reported, to unprecedented public commentary, critique, excitement, and previously unseen adulation of some of the more forthright practitioners. One of these early cases was an operation performed by Harry Windsor at St Vincent's Hospital in Sydney. The procedure was immediately successful but unfortunately the patient survived only a few weeks. Sadly, this became the usual experience and over the course of several months all of the original cohort of recipients died. The bubble had burst, enthusiasm turned mostly to condemnation, and even the motivation of many of the surgeons was questioned.

For all practical purposes transplantation was abandoned for several years although Barnard and Shumway continued their research. Eventually they prevailed and with the discovery and use of the safer, more effective immunosuppressive drug cyclosporin in the 1980s, cardiac transplantation became a practical and effective though expensive treatment.

I played no further part in these developments. Eventually, after some turgid politicking, St Vincent's Hospital was nominated as the site for the New South Wales heart transplant centre. Their results have been better than most and they now support a fine research department. In the beginning it was difficult to see how cardiac transplantation might turn out. Many of the inherent problems remain: it is extremely expensive, there will never be sufficient donors to make a major impact on population health, but, when it is successful it usually gives excellent long-term symptomatic improvement. Success has spawned even more adventurous transplantation efforts, such as lung transplantation, combined heart and lung transplantation, liver and other organ transplantation which in their turn have proven very effective for individual patients.

So there is the answer which I give to people when they ask if I have done many heart transplants: "Yes, I did a few but they were all done on pigs."

Coronary bypass graft

Was our coronary bypass graft at Prince Alfred Australia's first? How did we come to perform it? As is so often the case, the answer includes elements of luck, previous experiences, teamwork, and technical competence.

One Sunday in 1969 I was browsing through a recently arrived *American Journal of Cardiology* and happened upon the report from René Favaloro of the Cleveland Clinic describing his first series of coronary artery saphenous vein bypass graft operations. [The saphenous vein runs beneath the skin from the ankle to the groin and can readily be used as an arterial substitute.] Favaloro's paper was relevant to the case I was scheduled to operate that week at Royal Prince Alfred Hospital. Several background experiences are relevant to this story…

Back in 1963, the week before I started work with Michael DeBakey's team in Houston, Dr Ed Garrett had run into trouble with a cardiac operation. At the end of an open heart procedure Garrett could not wean the patient from cardiopulmonary bypass because the heart was not contracting adequately. As a last resort, Garrett harvested a length of saphenous vein from the patient's thigh and used it to form a graft from the ascending aorta to the left anterior descending coronary artery. The previously poorly contracting left ventricle recovered and the operation could be completed without further incident. By the time I joined the team the patient was well on the way to recovery, still being treated with kid gloves. The full implications of this excellent rescue were not fully understood at the time, but it must have begun to trigger Garrett's imagination.

Whatever the reason, Garrett was becoming interested in the Vineberg operation. Arthur Vineberg of Montreal had enjoyed some success with mobilising the left anterior thoracic artery, usually known to surgeons as the left internal mammary artery, "LIMA" from the inner chest wall, dividing its lower end, and implanting the bleeding end into a tunnel within the left ventricular muscle mass, in the hope of forming some anastomoses, or connections, with the native coronary arteries of the abnormal segment, so augmenting the local blood supply.

Peter Theile and I were tasked by Garrett to perform a series of experiments in the animal laboratory, in which we substituted a vein graft segment for the internal mammary artery, anastomosing one end of the vein to the descending thoracic aorta and implanting the other end into the left ventricular muscle, as in Vineberg's technique. The vein graft was readily available and versatile. It could be used to reach any area of the ventricular mass, potentially making it more adaptable than the internal mammary artery which at that time was seen as difficult to dissect, rather slender, and only long enough to reach the anterior wall of the left ventricle. Peter and I had some success with our experiments although many of the vein grafts later thrombosed.

Later in 1963 DeBakey hosted a visit by the pioneering cardiologist from Cleveland, Dr Mason Sones. Among his many achievements, Sones had refined the equipment and technique of cineangiography and applied them to cardiac imaging and diagnosis. During one of his angiographic procedures, he noted with horror that the catheter meant to deliver radio-opaque dye into the aorta had slipped into the mouth of a coronary artery. Direct injection of the dye into a coronary artery had previously been considered a death sentence for the patient. In this case the patient survived and the resulting angiogram showed the anatomy of the coronary artery system with hitherto unimagined clarity. Sones began studying patients with coronary arterial disease in a way that had never before been possible, allowing him to confirm or rule out coronary occlusive disease as the cause of the patient's symptoms by providing a precise anatomical and functional picture. Using this information, Sones and his surgical colleague Dr Donald Effler could now contemplate operating on selected cases.

In 1965, while I was working in the cardiac catheterisation laboratory at the Mayo Clinic, Giancarlo Rastelli arranged that he and I, along with his cardiologist friend Tasso Tsakiris, would visit the Cleveland Clinic to see Mason Sones' and Don Effler's work, specifically coronary angiography and cardiac re-vascularisation.

We travelled to Cleveland by Greyhound bus. During our transit in Chicago we saw the new movie *"Dr Zhivago"* but we had to leave for our onward overnight coach journey before the final scenes. Next day we were made welcome at the Clinic. Mason Sones was one of the great medical innovators of the 20th century. He was a hyperactive dynamo, another of those rare people who needs little sleep. He spent his life in his basement catheter laboratory assessing his patients, clarifying their diagnosis, and refining his equipment.

By the time we visited he was pioneering very different techniques and philosophy from those we were accustomed to at Mayo. Rather than using large-film biplane angiography, Sones had opted exclusively for single plane cineangiography, which provided good moving images, although not as clear as we were used to. But the versatility of his cine equipment allowed him to take multiple exposures during repeated selective injections of the radiopaque dye. He relied almost exclusively on those moving pictures to give him both anatomical detail and functional information and had scrapped the cumbersome historical diagnostic baggage of oximetry and indicator dilation curves. Because of the expense of the angiographic equipment, he had set up his laboratory in a large square area with preparation rooms on four surrounding sides. A Fellow, or junior doctor, was busy in each of those rooms dissecting a patient's brachial artery at the elbow. Sones would then take the patient into the lab, insert his catheter through an incision in the artery, perform the diagnostic procedure, and have the patient wheeled back to the preparation room for repair of the artery and suture of the skin, meanwhile studying a fresh patient from another preparation room. This mass production setup allowed him to study many more patients in the time that would have been taken in a conventional facility.

During our visit to the operating rooms we saw Don Effler and his team perform both of the operations which he was evaluating at that time. Guided by Sones' angiograms he could identify a part of the ventricle that was poorly supplied with blood and target that area for implantation of his Vineberg internal mammary artery graft. Results were reasonable and some patients enjoyed significant improvement of their symptoms. The post-operative angiograms also showed that some of the Vineberg grafts had formed significant anastomotic connections to join up with the coronary artery system beyond its site of blockage.

Of all the numerous patients being studied, a small subset had localised severe narrowing of one of the coronary arteries near its origin. Effler had standardised his method of supporting the patient on cardiopulmonary bypass while laying open the narrowed segment of the coronary artery. That incision was then closed with a patch of saphenous vein carefully sized so that it would bulge out and increase the diameter of the lumen or bore, relieving the obstruction without removing the obstructive atheromatous plaque, the fatty cholesterol deposit which had caused the narrowing. The Cleveland team referred to this domed patch as the Vistadome operation, after the observation coach on scenic American trains. This patch graft technique was widely used in renal and carotid artery surgery by that time, and, in the few cases in which it could be performed, it was a logical and effective operation.

Gian, Tasso and I returned to Rochester with much to ponder.

Which returns me to my Sunday reveries in 1969…

Dr Louis Bernstein had referred his patient with a recommendation that he would be suitable for a Vineberg operation. The patient was a clergyman in his mid-40s, incapacitated by angina pectoris; that is pain from the heart caused by inadequate blood supply to portion of his left ventricle. He was in many ways an ideal candidate, conscientious, a former distance runner, previously somewhat overweight but now slim and otherwise healthy. Our angiograms were good enough to show severe narrowing of the left anterior descending coronary branch just beyond its origin, with a relatively disease-free segment beyond the blockage.

I phoned Lou and proposed that this was a suitable case for Favaloro's new operation. The basic techniques were readily available to us. I was very familiar with the use of saphenous vein graft, by then the standard technique for dealing with narrowing of the femoral artery in the thigh. We discussed the idea with the patient, describing what we hoped to achieve and not hiding the fact that we were relying on reputable reports from overseas, although we had no local experience. The patient agreed and we went ahead.

The operation was straightforward. Anaesthesia was uneventful. I removed a segment of saphenous vein from his thigh, tied the small branches that were encountered, inflated it with heparinised saline and checked it for leaks or imperfections. After exposing the heart I inserted cannulae and began cardiopulmonary bypass with the heart-lung machine. This allowed the heart to empty and relax so that it was easy to expose the little coronary artery on the left front wall of the heart. By that time I had been using magnifying loupes [small telescopes mounted in a spectacle frame and focussed at a comfortable working distance] for most of my fine work. It was not difficult to make a clean incision in the relatively healthy part of the artery beyond the obstruction and attach the bevelled end of the saphenous vein to it, using Effler's technique of placing about 10 interrupted fine braided sutures around the lips of the incision, passing the stitches through the corresponding points in the vein, and tying them down carefully one by one. We did not at that time have the very fine monofilament sutures which later made this so much easier. The vein was trimmed to a comfortable length and anastomosed [sewn] to the front wall of the aorta. When the clamps were removed and blood was allowed to flow into the normal part of the coronary artery the heart immediately recovered, and we were able to withdraw the support of the heart-lung machine with no trouble. The post-operative course was uneventful.

The patient was soon awake and announced that his cardiac pain was gone. Heart surgeons have since heard this thousands of times. "It is like turning off a light switch" the patients say.

This young man had a good long-term result, typical of that which we came to expect. He returned to his parish and was active for many years, until the underlying arterial disease progressed and his angina pain returned. Louis repeated his angiogram study to confirm this progression and, interestingly, showed that my original graft remained open and apparently free of disease. With the help of my colleague Sandy Grant, who was by now more experienced in coronary work than I was, we re-operated and performed additional grafts to two or three more of his coronary artery branches. Again he had a good result but eventually, more than 15 years after the original operation, required further help in the form of coronary artery dilatation and stenting. A satisfactory result one would have thought.

If you imagine that the above success story led to a flood of referrals and the rapid establishment of coronary revascularisation as a standard treatment for a very common and lethal disease you are mistaken. Referrals were very scanty and the patients were usually in an advanced stage of the disease, desperate for relief, and had often already suffered severe damage to their heart muscle with consequent heart failure. Even so, we managed our first 15 consecutive operations without a death.

With hindsight, we can understand why it took so long for coronary artery bypass graft (CABG, pronounced Cabbage) to become the established treatment. Physicians, particularly cardiologists, were the doctors who treated coronary artery disease and its manifestations of angina pectoris and myocardial infarction. These were leaders of the profession and applied their treatments with varying but limited success. Because none of the treatments corrected the underlying disease process of progressive obstruction of the coronary arterial blood flow, none of the therapies improved the prognosis.

An epidemic of coronary disease was sweeping the Western world affecting many of the population, particularly males. Sudden death at an early age was a commonplace occurrence. When myocardial infarction did not cause immediate death it was managed medically with high ongoing mortality. Survivors of the acute illness commonly had permanent heart failure and were subject to recurrent infarctions [heart attacks].

Individual cardiologists continued to treat the patients' symptoms to their best ability. This was their stock in trade and, from the cynical point of view, one might unfairly say that their incomes and reputation might be threatened by a curative operation. It did not turn out that way, as I will show below.

Surgeons continued to treat the few patients who were referred and their techniques and results gradually improved. Over the next several years major multi-centre trials were undertaken in the USA and Europe and began to show beyond doubt that direct revascularisation of the heart cured symptoms, reduced the likelihood of myocardial infarction, and prolonged life expectancy. Concurrently, surgical results were improving and in the course of a few years the survivors were themselves the best ambassadors for the operation; everyone seemed to know someone who had had successful coronary artery grafts. Finally the dam walls were breached and within a short time CABG became the most frequently performed major operation in the Western world. By that time, I was mostly concerned with paediatric work and played no significant part in the ongoing development of this operation.

Before long we had excellent data from all advanced countries detailing the outcome of many thousands of operations. Not surprisingly, Cleveland Clinic became and remains one of the outstanding contributors to this work.

Douglas Baird, one of our trainees who had returned from the Mayo Clinic, was the main driver of the program at Prince Alfred. He was a competent surgeon and an outstanding organiser and political fixer. He created a coherent surgical team who ably managed the flood of referrals, and their results were comparable to any. Similar advances occurred throughout Australia and our national results have been among the world's best.

There was no single cause for the cascading improvements in coronary surgery. Over time, general management of patients improved, cardiopulmonary bypass was refined and became safer, surgical instruments and materials such as special sutures were developed, and surgeons' use of optical magnification became routine. New generations of trainees polished their skills in Australia and abroad, and operations became more standardised and efficient. Still, the coronary operations were expensive and time-consuming, and required significant recovery and rehabilitation time.

Concurrently with the flowering of surgical coronary revascularisation, a less invasive technique had been introduced by Andreas Gruentsig, in Zurich. Charles Dotter of Portland, Oregon had developed special balloon catheters to dilate localised narrowing of the femoral arteries. Gruentsig invented much finer strong balloons with which he could forcibly dilate the diseased coronary segments. When successful, this relief of obstruction could arrest or even reverse the progression of a myocardial infarction. The tendency of the dilated segment to close down again was finally resolved by invention of an expandable metallic mesh tube or stent, which was introduced with the balloon and expanded to splint open the artery.

Balloon dilatation and stenting (percutaneous transluminal coronary angioplasty, PTCA) was most obviously useful for urgent treatment of impending or recent myocardial infarction. Because it could be deployed almost within the hour and potentially at any time of day or night, with less preparation and organisation than a surgical revascularisation, it was rapidly shown to be an effective short-term measure. Over a few years, with refinements of equipment and technique and wide dissemination of the skills and personnel, it became competitive for elective and semi-elective treatment of many cases which previously would have been managed surgically.

At the time of writing, in 2018, more patients are treated by PTCA than by open surgery, with generally excellent results. There is still legitimate contention about which groups of patients are best treated by which technique, an argument too complex to be dealt with here. The number of open operations has plateaued over the last 10 to 15 years while the number of balloon procedures continues to grow. Surgery is mostly used for complex cases, for those requiring other surgical treatments such as valve operations, or for those patients who have not received lasting relief from PTCA.

Cardiology has been transformed into a very busy specialty, held in the highest repute, attracting excellent young doctors, its practitioners' earnings beyond the bounds of avarice.

What I learned from the first coronary artery bypass graft

I have described this surgical case in some detail, including events leading up to it and later developments, because it illustrates many important truths about the evolution of medicine and surgery.

Innovations are often triggered by practical problem-solving. A doctor who is confronted with a case for which an answer must be found will seek possible solutions from many sources. These ideas rarely come "out of the blue". Much more frequently they build on one or more pre-existing pieces of knowledge, often by innovative combinations of previous ideas.

Edward Garrett's single patient in which he used a saphenous vein bypass graft to salvage the life of an individual patient might have caused these developments to evolve earlier, but some of the building blocks were not yet available. Basic vascular techniques including use of saphenous vein grafts as arterial substitutes were already routine, but it took several years to develop the special sutures and techniques which we now use.

The work at Cleveland Clinic which we observed on our brief visit in 1965 helped bring these themes together. Increasing sophistication of angiographic imaging of the coronary arteries greatly clarified our understanding of the anatomical and functional implications of atheromatous disease. Early efforts at improving collateral blood flow to the heart culminated in the somewhat effective Vineberg operation, and Effler's direct Vistadome operations on localised obstructions were logical and effective in suitable cases.

"Chance favours the prepared mind" wrote Louis Pasteur. In this case, I had no difficulty in immediately seeing the applicability of René Favaloro's paper to my prospective patient, the young preacher. It was equally obvious to the patient's cardiologist and to the patient himself when frankly and clearly explained.

The operation was technically successful, reflecting our team's competence at that time.

This case was a beautiful example of the spectacular results usually achieved by this logical and effective method of improving coronary artery blood supply. Immediate relief of angina pain, followed by sustained improvement over many years are usual. Not surprisingly, the operation of itself does nothing to halt the progress of the underlying arterial disease and, over time, blockage of other coronary artery sites may cause recurrence of symptoms. Indeed, the same process that caused the coronary artery disease often attacks the vein grafts, causing them to narrow and fail. That is no longer necessarily the case: since that time far better medical interventions often retard the progress of arterial (and graft) disease. Cessation of smoking, control of blood pressure and diabetes, and statin drugs to reduce cholesterol levels are among the effective measures. Even when the disease progresses and symptoms return, repeat treatment is quite feasible with excellent results. These secondary procedures include further surgery or percutaneous angioplasty and stenting.

This story also illustrates the inertia in organised Medicine. Good results are not necessarily rewarded by more numerous referrals. Doctors are often temperamentally conservative, somewhat complacent about their traditional treatments, and potentially inhibited by their vested interests. Publication and promulgation of results has built-in delays. With time momentum builds, the word spreads in medical and lay circles and success speaks for itself.

The trickle of patients grew to a flood, surgeons everywhere responded to the challenge with better organisation, concentrated training, refinement of techniques and management, and the flowering of numerous excellent departments. A little later, but even more spectacularly, the growth of PTCA complemented, reinforced and partially replaced our surgical efforts.

Open heart surgery in infants and neonates

Open heart surgery was not consistently safe or effective for infants during its first 10 or 15 years.

Even before cardiopulmonary bypass was introduced, some congenital cardiovascular conditions were successfully treated with no need to open the heart. Persistent ductus arteriosus [in which a normal opening between the aorta and the pulmonary artery failed to close as usual after the baby's birth] was either ligated or else divided and the ends sutured. Coarctation (severe narrowing) of the aorta was managed by temporary clamping, excision of the narrow segment and re-anastomosis.

More complex intracardiac lesions could be palliated indirectly, usually by adjusting the pulmonary blood flow. Where the flow was inadequate, as in tetralogy of Fallot, it was enhanced by anastomosing [joining] a subclavian artery to the pulmonary artery [Blalock's "blue baby" operation]. Alternatively, in ventricular septal defects or similar lesions where the blood flow to the lungs was excessive it could be throttled by adjusting a constricting tape around the main pulmonary artery. These procedures palliated or "cloaked" the functional abnormality, so postponing curative repair (pallium = Latin for cloak).

Early attempts at open-heart surgery on small children and infants were unsatisfactory and mortality rates were high. The small body size of the patients made cannulation and exposure difficult. The delicate hearts were easily bruised by retraction. We also suspected something in the apparatus or process of cardiopulmonary bypass was to blame. These complex physiological abnormalities, collectively referred to as systemic inflammatory response syndrome, SIRS, were not understood for several more years. We also lacked effective long-term intensive care and ventilation to provide support during healing and recovery.

Over the years we accumulated several insights which helped us solve this problem:

- At normal body temperature a patient can usually recover from up to four minutes of arrested circulation without significant damage to the brain or other organs.

- Reducing body temperature to approximately 30C doubles this "safe" period.

- When body temperature is reduced much below 30C the risk of ventricular fibrillation or cardiac arrest becomes prohibitive; to achieve these deeper levels of hypothermia some form of artificial external support of the circulation is required.

- Frank Mills became interested in Charles Drew's report in 1959 of an ingenious technique of open-heart surgery which bypassed both the left and the right heart but continued to perfuse [pump blood] and ventilate the patient's own lungs in lieu of an artificial oxygenator. Without the need of an artificial lung, the body temperature was reduced to 20C or less, sufficiently cool for the circulation to be stopped for half an hour or more. After the repair was complete the procedure was reversed and the patient rewarmed using the extracorporeal pump circuit. Drew had good results in tetralogy ["blue baby] surgery. Frank and I established the Drew technique's feasibility in the animal laboratory but because it involved complex cannulation the method was not very satisfactory for small subjects. Other complications led to this method being abandoned and largely forgotten.

- Brian Barratt-Boyes in Auckland was encouraged by reports from Japanese colleagues, both in Japan and in Oregon, USA, of surgery using deep hypothermia. He reasoned that the exposure to cardiopulmonary bypass should be minimised by preliminary cooling in an ice bath, restricting the period of cooling bypass to a few minutes to complete the process. Similarly, during rewarming, a brief period of bypass was sufficient to restart the patient's circulation, completing the process in a warm water bath. Brian's results were better than had previously been recorded and we were seriously interested, but daunted by the complexity of this management.

• I was on sick leave for several months in late 1969. On my return I was asked to operate on a girl with "Scimitar Syndrome", a well understood but rare abnormality in which all the blood from the right lung, instead of draining to the left atrium, flowed through a large vein piercing the diaphragm to join the inferior vena cava, in this case within the liver (The big descending vein made a scimitar-shaped shadow on the chest X-ray). In principle we could place a baffle to subdivide the inferior vena cava to redirect the pulmonary vein blood through a natural or surgically created atrial septal defect into the left atrium, restoring normal circulation. The challenge was to isolate and control the large veins within the liver – theoretically possible but practically difficult and hazardous. At the Mayo Clinic I had occasionally deputised for John Kirklin to collaborate with the neurosurgeons to repair intracranial aneurysms. We would expose the heart, cannulate the right atrium and the aorta, and use the heart-lung machine and its heat exchanger to induce profound hypothermia. Neurosurgeon Colin McCarty had time to perform the neurosurgical procedure with circulatory arrest. The circulation was re-established with cardiopulmonary bypass to rewarm the patient. I resolved to use a similar technique for my Scimitar patient and it proved safe, simple and effective. A difficult and hazardous operation had been rendered safe and easy.

Anaesthetist John Overton and I synthesised these many experiences, using cardiopulmonary bypass with a heat exchanger to induce profound hypothermia before arresting the circulation for up to about 40 minutes, time enough to correct complex lesions in small patients, even new-borns. It proved effective. Success depended on simplicity, very thorough cooling of the brain and other body tissues over a period of at least 20 minutes, and meticulous care of cooling and re-warming rates to avoid bubble formation in the blood. With the heart empty and relaxed and the operative field free of cannulae and other clutter, it was possible to expose, visualise and correct the abnormalities in a way that had never been possible before, minimising handling, retraction and trauma of the heart tissues.

This simplified technique proved very effective and we achieved excellent results in ventricular septal defect, tetralogy of Fallot, transposition of the great arteries, and many other conditions in which early operation avoided long-term deterioration of the circulation. The time limitation required disciplined and organised operative planning and execution and imposed an ultimate restriction on the complexity of abnormalities which could be managed. Many surgeons were uncomfortable with the time pressures imposed upon them, and teaching less experienced trainees was a challenge.

Over time, all bypass equipment including the oxygenator, tubing, cannulae, and instruments have been specialised and miniaturised for the smaller patients. Largely under the stimulus of coronary artery surgery, improved suture materials became available along with microsurgical instruments to manipulate them. Much better magnifying glasses and lighting contributed to the technique. Concomitant improvements in intensive care and physiological management completed this evolution, allowing more complex operations to be performed without the need for long periods of circulatory arrest. The deep hypothermia with circulatory arrest principle is still useful in selected cases, particularly aortic arch surgery in which the relative simplicity and freedom from complex cannulation can be advantageous.

The magic of heart surgery

Surgery is a serious business engaged in by serious people and carries serious consequences.

It has been a privilege to be a small cog in the development of open-heart surgery during its first 50 years. Plenty of challenges remain: intellectual, scientific, diagnostic, technical, physical, ethical and emotional.

The background intellectual challenge is to master all the relevant information, keeping it front of mind and usable at all times. This encompasses the evolution of scientific knowledge of normal and abnormal structure and function of the heart and circulation, intimate knowledge of the principles and practice of cardiopulmonary bypass, and a complete and up-to-date mastery of one's own experiences, interpreted in light of the world's literature. This huge knowledge base is dynamic, ever-changing, and growing at a bewildering pace.

Accurate and precise diagnosis is fundamental to surgical planning and success. We are always in debt to our medical Cardiology and Anaesthesia colleagues for their skills, and equally to the scientists and engineers who have progressively refined and perfected the diagnostic techniques, machines and instruments. In the 1950s diagnosis was largely reliant on clinical history, physical examination including auscultation [listening] with a stethoscope, chest x-rays, and electrocardiogram. These diagnoses were and still are often surprisingly accurate and useful but, to achieve the precision required for consistent safe surgical repair, usually need to be enhanced by cardiac catheterisation and, increasingly, angiographic imaging. Catheterisation provides physiological measurement of pressures within the heart and estimates of blood flows from which resistances are derived.

Medical imaging presents us with essential pictures of the heart and other structures. Because blood casts a similar x-ray shadow to the heart and other fleshy tissues, angiography depends on rapid injection of a radio-opaque iodine-containing dye into the bloodstream while recording radiographic images. Selective injection of the dye through a cardiac catheter provides much more accurate information with less radiopaque medium. Two main recording systems have vied for supremacy in capturing the images. Large film changers handled sheets of x-ray film like a printer, exposing up to 6 or 12 frames per second, providing sharp images but no immediate representation of movement. Cine-angiography captures the images on film, at first 16mm but increasingly 35mm. Refinements in power of the x-ray sources, optics and film speed gave ever increasing improvement in image quality. Digital image capture has now supplanted film.

Echocardiography relies on the reflection and recording of sound waves from the heart structures (more correctly from the interfaces between adjacent structures). With further sophistication, this equipment displays two-dimensional moving pictures of virtual "slices" through the heart. These images, recorded on video and soon enhanced by Doppler representations of the movement, velocity and direction of blood flow through the heart, provide hitherto unachievable structural and functional information. [When a sound wave is reflected from a receding or approaching structure or blood cell the pitch or frequency appears to change, like the altered pitch of a passing train whistle. Comparison of the transmitted signal and its reflection provides an accurate assessment of the direction and velocity of the blood flow and can be measured or displayed as a real-time video image.]

Radioactive scanning techniques are useful in selective cases, particularly in assessing perfusion (blood flow) of particular areas of the heart muscle.

Magnetic Resonance Imaging (MRI) provides outstanding information about some of the more complex structural relationships.

Acquisition, display and interpretation of these images is primarily the responsibility of Cardiologists, Radiologists, and Nuclear Medicine experts but the surgeon needs complete confidence in their findings. Having integrated this wealth of diagnostic information, it is the surgeon's responsibility to formulate an operative strategy, assess the risks and potential benefits, and seek the consent of the patient and family before proceeding.

Cardiac surgeons are seldom the first port of call for patients and families. More likely, their primary care doctors have suspected a problem or an emergency has occurred, the case has been assessed in great detail by a cardiologist, and the possibility of surgery will have been raised in the earlier consultations. Ideally, a preoperative consultation will lay out the diagnosis as clearly and simply as possible, avoiding jargon. Sometimes simple diagrams are helpful. It is essential to state clearly what is the likely outcome without surgery, to describe the proposed procedure, including the risks of death or complications, and to voice the uncertainties.

Because they are mentally prepared for this discussion, patients and families usually agree. These formal consultations are the foundation for a proper moral contract between the parties, establishing a sound basis for an ethical bond. They also meet legal requirements for Informed Consent. Not least, the discussions establish trust, goodwill and support for those inevitable times when things do not turn out as planned.

Basic surgical technique is a learned skill: there are few if any born surgeons. If a trainee has any aptitude they can master the fundamentals quite quickly and become competent assistants. Over many hundreds of hours the manual skills fall into place and more muscle memory – more properly neuromuscular memory – is acquired. It really takes many thousands of hours before technique becomes almost automatic. The tricks and local knowledge, sometimes called heuristics, take years to acquire.

The operation proper affords further challenge. Much of the complexity is handled by near-ritualistic standardisation of techniques and procedures. Operating theatre layout, staffing, and communications fall into this category. The team assembles, necessary instructions and clarifications are made, anaesthesia and monitoring are established, and the routines of hand scrubbing, gowning and gloving, skin preparation and draping of the patient and preparation of the equipment soon become almost a matter of habit. The operation requires high alertness, although many surgeons, including myself, try to maintain an image of relaxed composure when possible. The operation usually goes according to plan but surprise and catastrophe are ever-possible. The procedure, especially in small children, infants and neonates, tests the extremes of human perception and performance. Even with optical magnification and the best available lighting, we frequently approach the limits of vision and manipulation and we are limited to available materials and instruments. Effective coordination and communication with other team members is an art in itself.

Cardiac operations are lengthy and demanding, conducted with intensity and often under time limitations; they are physically exhausting and emotionally stressful. While it is important to maintain an outward picture of assuredness and confidence, the risk of failure is ever top of mind. Any error in diagnosis, planning, or execution of an operation is likely to be fatal and not all errors are preventable or correctable.

The responsibility is grave and the burden of discussing failures with the surviving family members is heavy. Their response depends to some extent on their own philosophies of life but it can be eased to some extent by honest discussion at the time. A delayed debrief after several weeks is worthwhile. I always tried to state clearly what was found, what was done, and if anything might have been done differently. Often it was possible to clarify questions, misconceptions or misplaced feelings of guilt on the part of the parents. The surgeon's burden of failure, frustration, guilt, inadequacy, or depression is his or hers to carry. Professional detachment helps and there is always another challenge tomorrow. It is not for everyone.

The occasional agony of failure is outweighed most of the time by the relief, almost elation, of successful execution of a challenging operation. It is no small thing to deliver good news about a successful outcome, and the gratitude of patients and families is a huge reward. Even 30 or 40 years later, I often have patients write or phone or visit to express their thanks.

This chapter is my view of the challenges of clinical cardiac surgery as seen through the eyes of the surgeon. Here is a good place to acknowledge and emphasise the role of the patients and their families, the tremendous debt to teachers and colleagues, to the researchers who have so freely shared their knowledge and insights, to colleagues in Cardiology, Anaesthesia, Theatre and Ward Nursing, and Technicians, and to the administrators and even the politicians and philanthropists who have funded this work. Above all, it is appropriate to acknowledge the support of our own family members who forego so much of their own care and welfare in support of the demands of the surgeon's work.

Appendix 2: Administration and management

Politics

Medical politics is too important to leave to politicians. Many doctors believe they lack the time, temperament, or inclination to indulge in so grubby a pursuit. But we do know much more about Medicine than any nurse, administrator, or professional politician. This special knowledge uniquely equips us to represent our own best interests and to advocate for those of our patients, as well as contribute to the broader political discussion about priorities, asset allocation, and ethical values.

On returning from advanced training in USA in 1966 I became Staff Specialist at RPAH, and the next year was also seconded to the Children's Hospital. There were then very few salaried clinicians in New South Wales. Most of the doctors directly employed by hospitals were laboratory people – Pathologists, Haematologists, Radiologists, plus a few Anaesthetists. Almost all of the Physicians and Surgeons at the major teaching hospitals served in an honorary capacity giving their time, clinical services and teaching pro bono, in recognition of the status of their appointments. They made their living from private practice in their consulting rooms and at private hospitals. Viewed in hindsight this is a bizarre arrangement, sometimes described by the wits as a "Robin Hood" arrangement whereby the doctors robbed the rich and gave to the poor. Whatever its defects, it provided the indigent patients with free access, if they were lucky, to the most distinguished doctors in the land. It cannot be denied that it was a "two tier system", too good to escape the attention of socialist do-gooders. See below.

Specialties such as mine demanded full time commitment, especially in their developmental phases. To put the matter simply, without some salary, regardless of its source, I could not have provided this full-time service. In

1966 the salaries offered were not very generous, reflecting the low standing of those providing support services in the hospital, and perhaps in recognition of the relative security of a full-time government-funded job.

There had been disputation about which industrial body should represent the hospital Staff Specialists. Many of the leading hospital administrators insisted that we, like them, be represented by the Public Service Association, a large group encompassing all public servants in the State. Some of the medical salaried hotheads insisted on forming their own Public Medical Officers Association (PMOA), feeling, probably correctly, that we could better represent ourselves despite our small numbers instead of relying on the support of the much larger union, most of whose members were employed in clerical or administrative roles.

There was, and is, a technical difference between a Union, normally associated with tradespeople and labourers, and a professional Association such as ours or the much bigger Australian Medical Association. Nevertheless, the role of the PMOA was to put forward our case for adequate remuneration and conditions of work, if necessary litigating in the industrial courts for the purpose.

I contributed for many years to this effort, representing my hospital on the Association's Committee of Management. Early on, during appearances at the Industrial Court, I gave evidence as to the length of training, degree of skill, complexity and responsibility which clinicians brought to the job, and which, we contended, required recognition in the form of a professional salary and conditions.

By 1972 the juicy prize of socialised medicine was well in the sights of the up-and-coming politician Gough Whitlam. Among his numerous ambitious, sometimes desirable, sometimes crazy, and the often mutually incompatible components of "The Program", was a huge shakeup of Health and Medicine, resulting in something akin to the British National Health system. The archaic Honorary medical system would certainly have to go. Doctors would lose their professional independence and become salaried public servants, patients would do what they were told, and presumably private medical practice would be outlawed.

Many Australian doctors had personal experience of the British system, having taken advanced training there. The English Minister who introduced it, Aneurin Bevan, had reportedly said of medical opposition soon after World War II: "I will stuff their mouths with gold". The system was introduced without too much fuss but there were many shortcomings. It was expensive, patients had no choice whatever, even in their choice of general practitioner, there was no financial incentive for hard work or improvement, little effective competition, and some of the less motivated people gave less than full-hearted value for their money. We did not welcome a fully socialised arrangement for Australia and had no intention of meekly accepting it.

The Australian Medical Association resisted the proposed scheme with some success. The AMA, as an Association, probably could not and chose not to strike, rightly considering their duties to the patients overrode considerations of personal gain. No such scruples inhibited the politicians. In the event, Whitlam's General Practice component, called Medibank, was enacted, essentially as a government funded remuneration of General Practitioners on a fee for service basis, paying 85 per cent of a supposed "most common fee" for each attendance, with the patient expected to provide the small balance if they could. The GP could, if they chose, accept the government payment only, billing the government directly and saving some administrative costs. This messy arrangement, having some good and some bad features, persists largely unchanged to this day. The famously incompetent Whitlam Government lost office in 1975 and the implementation of the hospital component, later called Medicare, had to await the Hawke government in 1983.

With the looming Socialisation of hospital Medicine, there was a serious political problem. As explained above, the AMA was to some extent hobbled in its industrial capacity by not being a Trade Union. The PMOA was also not a Union and in any case represented salaried staff and so could hardly have acted for the threatened Honorary Medical Officers. The specialist Colleges such as the Royal Australasian College of Surgeons and the Royal Australian College of Physicians and various others had been advised that any overt political activity would void their charitable status and hence their tax-exempt privilege.

Somewhat helter-skelter, bodies such as the Australian Association of Surgeons were cobbled together as overt industrial bodies, ready to take the fight to the Government. It was a textbook example of "divide and rule", with the profession nominally represented by half a dozen organisations, many of them inhibited either by their constitution or by their own ethics or anxieties, some more committed to General Practice than specialist hospital practice, and few of their members with much stomach for a fight with the rampant Socialists.

I was elected as representative of the Society of Cardiothoracic Surgeons to the Australian Association of Surgeons, who along with the Australian Orthopaedic Association and the Australian Society of Anaesthetists largely led the opposition against the wholesale socialisation of hospital practice. This politically militant activity was unfamiliar and uncomfortable for most of us. Our main leaders were Bruce Shepherd, an Orthopaedic Surgeon who had overthrown the leadership of the AMA because of its perceived weakness and its appetite for capitulation, Michael Aroney, of the AAS, a loquacious General Surgeon, and Peter Catts, a colourful figure who soon became an important advocate for development of a private hospital system of comparable strength to the public system.

Seemingly endless meetings were held, occupying most of every weekend and mainly conducted at the Sydney Airport Hilton Hotel for the convenience of fly-in fly-out delegates. Discussions were verbose and sometimes confusing but a few consistent themes emerged. The so-called Procedural Specialists (Surgeons, Anaesthetists, Orthopaedic Surgeons, Urologists, O & G, et cetera) were implacably opposed to a United Kingdom style Socialised arrangement, they would not accept compulsory salaried service for professionals, and they were determined to preserve some form of private practice, free of price fixing.

Governments were unreceptive to good faith negotiation. The New South Wales Health Minister, Ron Mulock, was affectionately known by his boss, Premier Neville Wran, as Meathead. The Commonwealth Health Minister of the day was the intelligent, self-satisfied, voluble and doubt-free Neal Blewett.

The mood within the profession became increasingly ugly and the Orthopaedic Surgeons, led by Bruce Shepherd, resigned en masse from the public hospital system. After some time, most of the remaining procedural specialists resigned or threatened to do so. Wran was sufficiently outraged to lose his legendary political judgement, irrationally threatening not only to replace all of those who had resigned by imports from overseas, but to legislate that no one who had resigned would ever again work in the New South Wales public system. This overreach incensed even the more moderate practitioners and waverers. For example, my group, the Cardiothoracic Surgeons, took a full-page advertisement in the broadsheet newspapers stating our intention to resign. In one of the well-publicised interchanges of that hectic time, Neville Wran sought the assurance of his friend Victor Chang, the cardiac surgeon from St Vincent's, that he would not go along with this threat. Victor, who was at that time the most high profile transplant surgeon in Australia and a protégé of Wran, announced publicly that he would resign along with his colleagues if necessary.

Things rapidly came to a head. A few cooler heads within the Labor movement prevailed on the Prime Minister Bob Hawke to convene a summit meeting in Canberra. On a stormy afternoon a dozen of us representing the various subgroups were flown to the Capital in some small charter aircraft. This group came to be known as the 12 apostles. A lengthy meeting in the Cabinet room, expertly chaired by PM Bob Hawke and including the Federal and State health ministers and senior bureaucrats, failed to achieve any resolution. There was essentially no way for the politicians to win, but there was no certainty as to what form a resolution might take.

Inexplicably, the Federal President of the Australian Medical Association, Lindsay Thompson, a GP with no mandate to negotiate on behalf of the profession at large, chose to capitulate, throwing away most of the political leverage which the New South Wales specialists had generated.

An uneasy peace was established. Medicare in its current form was enacted. The Honorary system was abandoned although some diehard militant Orthopaedic Surgeons maintained their version of it, accepting positions as Visiting Medical Officers (the term for what used to be Honorary Medical Officers) but refusing any payment for their services. Most of the former Honoraries eventually accepted posts as VMOs and were paid on an hourly basis. The few surgeons who previously had worked as salaried medical officers or as academic surgeons continued much as before. So, at considerable financial cost and irreparable destruction of goodwill, and with some perceived compromise of professional independence, the Surgeons and other Specialists had been notionally brought under some control of the political and administrative bosses.

One very good outcome of the messy "doctors' dispute" interlude was that several of the leading lights of the resistance moved quickly to establish a much better and bigger private hospital system than had existed before, and gave a significant amount of their time, talents and effort to perfecting these private hospitals. Another good outcome of the tensions of the time was the establishment and maturation of the Day-only surgery movement. Special units within existing hospitals and several freestanding private one-day surgery centres were established and proved to be popular, efficient, safe and cost effective.

With hindsight, one of the worst outcomes was the loss, probably forever, of the esprit de corps which had sustained the teaching hospital HMOs. Their leadership and clinical, teaching and administrative work which had been given freely in the past was effectively transferred to the new efforts within the private hospital system. Ill will generated by the brutal stand-off with the politicians persists and probably will continue for many years to come. Few of those who lived through those days will likely trust professional politicians. The politicians who had long envied the independent mindset and professional status of doctors may well have been satisfied with their outcome but the intangible costs were grave.

What I learned

Politics is indeed a dirty and distasteful game but should never be left to the politicians.

One of my most earnest but probably futile wishes is for senior clinicians to resume more of their traditional role in the management of hospitals.

Royal Alexandra Hospital for Children: Administration

Doctors are generally intelligent and ambitious and have a lively sense of their own importance. When I joined the staff of the Children's Hospital some of my new colleagues were among the few salaried medical officers, and also willing to participate in the low-level tugs-o-war within the institution.

Each major hospital had an active Medical Staff Association, distinct from the formal Hospital Administration but important in allowing some representation of the staff to the official management structure. Typically, there would be a monthly meeting of the staff, usually following dinner and a few drinks. Discussion was often enthusiastic, voluble, bombastic and somewhat irrational. But it was a good opportunity to let off steam.

In addition to the traditional tensions between Clinical Staff and Administration, historic changes were in train. Back then, many of the senior staff in our paediatric hospital were self-taught and often lacked formal credentials.

They might have been General Practitioners with a particular interest in Paediatrics who, through their enthusiasm and advocacy, were devoting a large part of their practice to care of children. But times were changing.

A younger generation of Physicians and Surgeons with formal training and qualifications in various specialties had been appointed. The distinguished Professor of Paediatrics, Dr (later Sir) Lorimer Dods, had gathered around him a coterie of specialists dealing with areas such as Paediatric Oncology, Thoracic Medicine, Endocrinology and Neurology, as well as formally qualified General Paediatricians.

A younger group of physicians, roughly of my age cohort, were coming online in areas such as Nephrology and Cardiology, and many of them were being employed either part-time or fully salaried.

On the surgical side, the senior staff were similarly stratified, with senior members holding specialist qualifications but not necessarily in Paediatrics. They were specialists such as Plastic Surgeons, Urologists and Orthopaedic Surgeons with a special interest in Paediatric practice.

Also some of the service specialties such as Pathology, Radiology and Anaesthesiology were becoming staffed largely or partly by salaried specialists.

This era of inevitable change was resisted by the usual human traits of inertia, self-interest, financial interest, professional and academic hubris, and the particular medical themes of competition for patients and resources. Staff meetings were usually exciting.

Decisions were formally reported through the General Superintendent (CEO) to the Board of Management but there was no obligation on the part of Management to respond. Administration seemed happy to accept this mechanism to relieve tension without ceding executive power to the Medical Staff.

Having participated in the Medical Staff Association for years, I was elected to replace my friend Denby Bowdler as Honorary Secretary after his death in an air crash in 1976.

My Chairman at that time was Arnold Tink, an Honorary Physician of conservative hue and a stickler for fairness and procedure. After some years I succeeded Arnold as Chairman.

The Chairman and Secretary of the Staff Association were invited ex officio to join the Board of Management, the senior management committee of the hospital.

Each month we met in the boardroom to deliberate over a typical Board agenda presented by the General Superintendent. Meetings were chaired by the President of the Hospital Board, the stockbroker Douglas Burroughs.

The Board included some senior medical staff, business people from the City, civic minded ladies who had supported the hospital financially and practically for many years, and the Matron, now called the Director of Nursing.

Discussions were somewhat formal, almost always civil, and usually led to consensual decisions, which in theory were to be carried out by the hospital executive.

The Board of Management delegated many of its deliberative functions to various subcommittees.

Some of the important committees on which I served were: –

Member, Medical Sub-Committee/ Medical Advisory Committee	1975 - 1998
Member, Theatre Management Committee	1980 - 1998
Chairman, Theatre Management Committee	1985 - 1996
Chairman, Clinical Cross-Infection Committee	1985 - 1993
Member, Patient Care Committee	1985 - 1996
Chairman, Patient Care Committee	1993
Member, Research Grants Committee	1993 - 1997
Member, Research Grants Advisory Committee	1988 - 1997
Member, Ethics Committee	1985 - 1998
Chairman, Ethics Committee	1994 - 1998
Member, Library Committee	1988 - 1996
Member, Audit Advisory Committee	1992 - 1996
Member, Budget Review Committee	1994

As the functions of these subcommittees evolved they took up more and more time. I was a willing participant because it was a chance to offer an informed clinical viewpoint to these discussions.

Following the retirement of Dr Douglas Cohen I was appointed Chairman of the Division of Surgery. The exact role of the Chairman was far from clearly defined, as the many subspecialties of Surgery were largely autonomous, each having its own notional Head. These Heads, in their turn, were often defined by their seniority or by their clinical distinction.

The Chairman's responsibilities included recruitment of new staff and general concerns of quality and standards, including standards of clinical care and general professional requirements. All these matters were carried out through poorly defined relationships with individual surgeons, department Heads, and the Hospital Management.

The Chairman of the Division also had sweeping but ill-defined responsibility for public relations and politics. These included representation of the surgeons within the hospital and interaction with other specialties, representation of Paediatric Surgery and its specialties within the broader Surgery community, and presenting a public face to the community at large.

Because of the loosely defined responsibilities and lines of command and communication, the Chairman's lot was often frustrating. On the other hand, the opportunity to work with a group of competent and highly motivated colleagues was both interesting and emotionally rewarding. I tried conscientiously to study the art of management but freely admit that I had little native ability for it. My main contribution seemed to be to see and be seen, and to be available for consultation, counselling, and general conflict resolution.

Chair of Paediatric Surgery

This chapter has been the most difficult to write of this entire memoir, for reasons which will become apparent.

In the earlier section of this book on my undergraduate education in paediatrics, I wrote warmly of Prof Lorimer Dods, a legendary teacher and outstanding character. Already an established and successful general practitioner and staff member of the Royal Alexandra Hospital for Children, he had become inaugural Professor of Child Health in 1949 when the chair was established jointly by the Faculty of Medicine of Sydney University and the Royal Alexandra Hospital for Children. In the same year Dods had been named Director of the new Institute of Child Health, a joint endeavour of the Commonwealth of Australia, Sydney University and Children's Hospital.

After Lorimer's acclaimed reign as Professor he had been succeeded by Prof Tom Stapleton and later by Prof Kim Oates. Throughout this long and successful period there had been no accompanying Professor of Paediatric Surgery. Kim Oates, along with General Superintendent of the Children's Hospital, John Yu and the Dean of the Faculty of Medicine at Sydney University, Prof Richard Gye, resolved in the late 1980s that this deficiency should be corrected. When the Chair of Surgery was advertised, they "suggested" that I apply. In due course I was appointed inaugural Professor of Paediatric Surgery.

My time as professor was enjoyable in some ways but frustrating overall. I enjoyed the opportunity to teach, I was stimulated by the chance to supervise a few successful PhD candidates, and I continued my role as Head of the Division of Surgery within the hospital, much as before. Where I failed was in getting sufficient support, including financial support. Also, there was a general lack of enthusiasm within the existing surgical staff for research and I was not successful in recruiting many young associates for this purpose. On reflection, I was probably not the right person for the job, the position was not fully resourced, and I was over-extended clinically, administratively and politically. In truth, I was not cut out for this particular job, and probably should have thought more deeply before taking it on.

Building the New Children's Hospital at Westmead

The original Sydney Hospital for Sick Children opened in an old school building in Glebe in 1880. By the turn of the century it had become inadequate for its growing workload, and a new site was secured on Pyrmont Road, Camperdown.

Funds were raised by public subscription and the foundation stone was laid in 1903. The following year the Queen, Alexandra, bestowed her name on the institution – the Royal Alexandra Hospital for Children. The first buildings were opened in 1907. These solid administrative and ward blocks remained in use for 90 years. According to need and available funding, numerous additional buildings of varying distinction were constructed on the Camperdown campus. Necessary modifications to render existing ward structures fit for modern purposes were restricted by the weight-bearing brick walls and inflexible floor plans. Although the old place was held in strong affection by most staff members, there was no gainsaying the near Dickensian standard of some of our physical facilities.

By the 1970s some enthusiasts, especially Don Gengos, had begun to promote the idea that a new hospital might be built as a Centenary project to be opened in 1980, but nothing came of it. Nevertheless, caseloads grew, and evolving medicine and surgery required more and more specialised technical accommodation. Planning began for a possible "Medical Services Block" to be located behind the existing buildings fronting the Pyrmont Bridge Road. In the event these plans came to a dead end.

By the 1980s the State government became receptive to the concept of a new, much larger, modern hospital nearer the geographical centre of Metropolitan Sydney. The same problem had stimulated the construction of Westmead adult Teaching Hospital a few years earlier. When the Minister for Health suggested this to our Hospital Board I was one of the early supporters of General Superintendent, Dr John Yu and Chairman of the Board, Mr John Dunlop, who became early protagonists. We were conscious that these opportunities did not arise often, that resisting such essentially logical and reasonable ideas was unlikely to be fruitful, and that it was worth the considerable effort to overcome the usual inertia. It is certainly difficult to leave a well-loved institution, especially when there are practical difficulties such as living or having consulting rooms in Camperdown or the Eastern part of the city.

After some discussion and dissension, the government made available the site of a former but now defunct Speedway, adjacent to the already established Westmead adult hospital, and planning began.

Our first hurdle was to break through the fixed thinking of those who had been planning a Medical Services Block for Camperdown. The brief was now much more extensive as we needed to create a comprehensive facility for all our present and future medical, surgical, inpatient, outpatient and ancillary needs. Serious committee work was now required to produce a good Functional Brief. This was a new concept to me, but I rapidly grasped the principle that "form follows function" [The phrase stems from Chicago architect Louis Sullivan, 1896, and was the principle animating the German Bauhaus design school between World Wars I and II]. The better one can specify the functional needs, the more practical and effective a building the architects can design. Planning is a serious task and requires open minds and painstaking work.

The state government needed to achieve some stimulatory spending to counteract a financial recession at the time. The Public Works Architect committed three different firms to design and build three pavilions which would be constructed side-by-side to comprise the new hospital. The result was an interesting mixture of styles. The Outpatients block employed a few quirky gimmicks to attract or distract the young patients. A Services and Inpatients' block included areas such as Operating rooms, Engineering, Administration, and Conference rooms, as well as Wards. An Office area comprised Specialist Departments including office and investigative areas. This eccentric plan resulted in an interesting building which was delivered on time and on budget for about $250 million – which seemed a fair amount of money at the time.

By 1995 the New Children's Hospital at Westmead was ready for us to move in. We slowed down activities in the old hospital to thin out our inpatient numbers. All the stuff we were moving was packed into small cartons which were transported very efficiently by swarms of small trucks on the appointed day.

There was a flurry to move in to the new quarters, reassemble everything, and tidy up before resuming full operations.

Perhaps predictably, at the time of publication in 2023, the hospital was undergoing redevelopment.

Domestic architecture footnote

About the time that we were engaged with planning of the new hospital, Marilyn and I reached a decision that we could rebuild our weekend cottage at Killcare with a view to living there for our retirement.

During a ski holiday we roughed out some of the ideas and on return to Eastwood I began to organise them into a proper functional brief using the word processing capabilities of my Apple II computer.

We enticed the Killcare architect, John McKinney, to join us for coffee on site. When John flourished his notepad and asked what we had in mind, we were able to produce our printed list of requirements. That gave him food for thought.

John did a good job of translating these functional needs into a very effective plan to utilise the attractive features of our site, especially the outlook over Hardy's Bay. We engaged the services of Laurie Smith, a Central Coast builder. Construction was slow, held back by persistent wet weather and later by the delayed supply of some important white goods. Laurie reckoned that the bathtub was being rowed from Germany. But when our weekend cottage was complete in 1995 it was so attractive that we moved in and made it our permanent home, commuting to Sydney a few days a week.

We lived in our Killcare house for over a quarter of a century. It met our design requirements and has served us well, an excellent "machine for living in" with few shortcomings. A good house, maybe quirky but very comfortable.

Council of Royal Australasian College of Surgeons

I was a member of the Council of the Royal Australasian College of Surgeons from 1991 through 1997 and served on many of its committees. The College was evolving in its functions, management and politics. Established in 1927 and modelled loosely on the American College of Surgeons and the various UK Royal Colleges, it sought to unite the surgical establishments of Australia and New Zealand. At that time most qualified Australian and New

Zealand surgeons had trained abroad, usually in the United Kingdom but sometimes elsewhere, and a few still were essentially General Practitioners with an interest in surgery. Among other things, the 1927 Memorandum of Association stated that the objectives for which the college was established were:

- To cultivate and maintain the highest principles of surgical practice and ethics
- To promote the practice of surgery under proper conditions by securing the improvement of hospitals and hospital methods
- To arrange for adequate postgraduate surgical training
- To promote research in surgery
- To bring together the surgeons of Australia and New Zealand periodically for scientific discussion and practical demonstration of surgical subjects
- To initiate and watch over and if necessary to petition Parliament or promote deputations in relation to measures affecting the College.

The Founders of the College briefly considered building its headquarters in the new Australian Capital City of Canberra but considered it impractical at the time. After squabbling for some time between Sydney and Melbourne, some said facetiously that they might have considered a houseboat on the River Murray, but eventually settled on Melbourne. That is about as central as you can get in the widespread territories of Australia and New Zealand. The fine pseudo-Georgian building that they erected there came to be seen as a clubby base for Melbourne General Surgeons and they made good use of it.

As surgical specialisation developed and spread, the relationships between the various subspecialties and the parent General Surgery organisation were maturing. During the Presidency of Tom Reeve, himself an Australian General Surgeon who had taken his postgraduate training in USA, he was conscious of significant tensions and keen to consolidate all surgical specialties under one umbrella. Members of small specialties with relatively few members rarely were elected to the governing Council; they lacked the necessary voting power. Reeve addressed this by establishing that smaller subgroups would each elect their own representative to Council, in addition to the broadly elected original Councillors. Melbourne Cardiothoracic Surgeon, Bruce Davis, was our first representative and I succeeded him.

Council meetings were held three times a year in Melbourne and once to coincide with the Annual Scientific Congress, wherever that was held. The usual agenda papers made an inch-thick packet, and subcommittee papers were even more voluminous. Enough to occupy most of the preceding Sunday, plus the Melbourne flight. I usually travelled to Melbourne on the Monday, occupied Tuesday and part of Friday with committee meetings, and spent the whole of Wednesday and Thursday in the Council meeting proper.

When it was convenient, Marilyn would accompany me on these trips as it was an excellent opportunity to meet the other surgical leaders and their families and to enjoy the many delights of Melbourne.

Council meetings were held in the impressive panelled Boardroom. The President sat at the head of the table flanked by his Treasurer on the right and the CEO, then called the College Secretary, on his left. About 20 counsellors were ranged around the long table, the more junior usually furthest "below the salt". The wall facing the President was filled by the huge bookcases of the marvellous Cowlishaw historical medical book collection. [The Cowlishaw Collection contains hundreds of historic books on medicine and related subjects, including many early, classic and rare editions. It was purchased in 1943 from the Estate of Dr Leslie Cowlishaw, a physician and bibliophile in Sydney. (Ref: Royal Australasian College of Surgeons website, 2018)]

The Councillors were an impressive and interesting group, leading surgeons near the peak of their careers, often in their 60s, prepared to devote weeks of their time every year to the cause. They were well motivated and almost unfailingly well informed, which is just as well because many of them were pretty garrulous. I mostly chose to sit quietly, listen and learn, intervening when something needed to be said or to make some critical point. A humorous interjection sometimes served the purpose. Office Bearers were elected every two years and their contribution to the affairs of the College was extraordinary. The President would often put his own Practice on hold for the duration because he not only had to preside at our meetings but also direct all the activities of the College, represent it at political and other professional bodies in Australia and New Zealand, and participate in the affairs of the International Colleges, especially those of the United Kingdom and USA.

Much of the routine work was entrusted to committees, with their findings being further discussed and hopefully endorsed by the Council proper. A few of the more interesting committees on which I served were: –

- General Scientific Meeting, later called the Annual Scientific Congress: This committee was responsible for the preparation and oversight of the important Annual General Meeting and its scientific component. This important event rotated through the Australian and New Zealand Capitals, and occasionally in one of the South-East Asian Capitals in recognition of the growing number of our Fellows in those areas.

- Education: Continuing Medical Education was becoming increasingly important. Surgical science, practice and technology, like all of Medicine, is rapidly evolving and demands ongoing learning from all of its practitioners.

- Library: As well as the Cowlishaw Collection mentioned above, the College building housed an impressive Library of surgical textbooks and periodicals, especially relating to General Surgery. It was a very valuable asset.

- Technology: President John Hanrahan asked me to chair a committee dealing with the rapidly increasing role of technology in surgery. With hindsight, we might have put more emphasis on the growing role of minimally invasive surgery and increasingly sophisticated imaging. In the event we concentrated more on the role of computers in practice and research and the growing interest in electronic communications. Interestingly, at this phase of development (early 1990s), computerisation in general and electronic communications in particular had only been embraced seriously by a minority of the Council members and of surgeons as a whole, and a surprising number of our brethren were cautious, sceptical, or even hostile. A few years later the Internet blossomed, "everybody" used email, and electronic databases came to dominate almost everything, including the medical literature. A few years after my departure, even the College Library is run almost entirely electronically. This time at least, my timing was not quite right.

- Research: College was and is a major financial supporter of Surgery research. Evaluation and grading of research proposals was a major task, time-consuming and demanding of concentration. To discriminate between the many applicants, most of whom had significant merit, could be difficult, and many worthwhile projects missed out on funding. The yield in high quality and relevant scientific output was reward enough for us.

- Working Party on Provision of Tertiary Medical Services to Pacific Island countries: (Pacific Island Project: P.I.P). As described above under Sydney Adventist Hospital Healthcare Outreach, I was co-opted to this project initiated by the Australian Government Department of Foreign Affairs to rationalise and consolidate several existing voluntary surgery services which it was funding in the Pacific, and which partnered with the Adventist Outreach activities to cover Cardiac Surgery.

Social activities

Those of us from out of town dined informally at one of Melbourne's excellent restaurants on Tuesday evenings, often choosing Lygon Street. During the full Council meeting we usually invited some distinguished guest to join us at noon, give an address to Council, and participate in discussion. In this way we benefited from the wisdom of numerous scientists, a few politicians, some artistic people, and industry figures who would then join us at lunch.

The evening between the two main Council meeting days was an opportunity for a friendly dinner of Council members, any of their partners who were available, and invited members of the lay staff of College, with proceedings usually enlivened by a wide-ranging address from one of our company.

Subsequent developments

In the 20 years since I served on Council, the College has grown, evolved and changed, surely for the better.

Around the turn of the Century it morphed into a grown-up tertiary education institution, embracing the medical education tropes of the day including formal curricula, structured supervised training, more formal documentation, and a more University-like examination system. This is all for the better but it has made many of the processes more cumbersome and expensive.

More recently, the institution has become more touchy-feely, with more emphasis on human factors, error and its avoidance, and “non-technical skills”. These include matters such as communication, technical impairment, discipline, practice management, business matters and the like. The latest preoccupation has been with bullying and harassment which, to nobody's surprise, occur as much within surgery as in any other endeavour.

Appendix 3: Travel — A detailed summary

Marilyn and I had dreamt of spending significant time and resources during our retirement seeing as much as possible of Australia and other parts of the world. Some memorable trips are described here.

Queensland by rail, 2002 and 2010

Our fortunate first choice was a one month's long trip through outback Queensland, guided by St James Rail. This tour company, of which we had learned while we were still overseas, was run by an interesting character called Owen Johnstone-Donnet. He is a lifelong rail enthusiast who got into the travel business while still a teenager, by organising weekend excursions for some of the parishioners at his Church. Subsequently he has worked as an aide to various politicians, including John Howard and Gladys Berejiklian. Owen is quite a remarkable fellow, large, round faced, well fed, very intelligent and articulate, helpful, calm, tactful, friendly, energetic and very effective. These are handy attributes for a tour guide; I have rarely seen him show signs of irritation or frustration in any situation.

That first Queensland trip made use of as many as possible of the remaining long-distance sleeper-train journeys, reaching as far inland as Mount Isa, Longreach, and Charleville. We were shadowed around Queensland by a comfortable coach which provided for all the missing links in current train timetables and tracks. When possible we took advantage of many remnant bits of rail track which are maintained by various enthusiastic voluntary groups running rail motors, steam trains, or even fettlers' jinkers on the old tracks [The fettlers who maintained the track used these little three or four wheel carts to transport themselves and their supplies along the rails. Propulsion was often by manpower using various rowing action mechanisms, even pedals, or simple petrol engines in Queensland. When a train approached, the fettlers used to tip the jinker off the track to let the train pass.]

Over a month we saw a huge area of Queensland and experienced overnight sleeper accommodation in the soon to be discarded long-distance trains.

A few years later, in 2010, we again travelled with St James Rail even further into outback Queensland, as far south-west as Birdsville, as far nor-west as the Barkly tablelands, and as far north on the coast as the Town of 1770 [so called to commemorate the visit of Captain James Cook's barque Endeavor in that year].

Queensland has a wealth of history, including the pastoral industry, mining, aviation, agriculture and exploration. Once you leave the coast, most of the areas are truly remote, thinly settled and with often very basic facilities. No matter, Owen and his crew gave marvellous service, solved all problems with tact and patience, and made a huge effort to keep everyone comfortable and interested.

Darwin to Perth by coach, 2004

Another St James Rail exploit was to fly to Darwin, spend a day or two there, then travel to Perth by coach, beginning at Kakadu, making the great sweep westward through Kununurra, Derby, through the inland part of the Kimberley to Broome, thence looping inland through the iron provinces of the Pilbara, returning to the coast around Karratha and then sticking mainly to the coast through the Exmouth Gulf area, Geraldton, and at last through the West Australian wheat fields to Perth. To complete this odyssey we travelled back to Sydney by the Indian Pacific train, one of our many trips on this line.

Car trips in Australia

We enjoyed many car trips long and short throughout Australia.

One memorable adventure was patterned on a pre-war trip that Marilyn had made as a child with her parents and sister, Roslyn, to visit her Uncle Fred when he was managing Drummond Slopes cattle Station near Alpha in Queensland. We had Marilyn's father Hector's original letters to his mother, in which he had described this camping trip in detail. Following the directions as closely as we could, we set off from Katoomba, through Bathurst, Dubbo,

Narromine and Nyngan and stayed the night in a motel on the south bank levee of the Darling River at Bourke. From there the route continued north into Queensland and through Cunnamulla, Charleville and Blackall, reaching Barcaldine in late afternoon. Every lodging in town was occupied by a convocation of all the Queensland Ford dealers. We turned smartly left and drove into the setting sun to find a good hotel in Longreach.

Next morning we retraced our tracks and headed east to Alpha, stopping at the pub for lunch. By chance we saw a large wall map in the Bar which showed all the old cattle stations of Queensland. We identified Drummond Slopes and decided to make a wide detour and try to find the property. From their turnoff we drove a long way towards the homestead but saw nothing except a herd of Longhorn cattle. The afternoon was slipping away and fuel running low, so we found a rough development road further south and followed it east to Springsure where there was fuel and lodging. The next day we resumed our trip, heading through the Blackwater coal province, reaching Rockhampton and Yeppoon to stay the night. This had also been visited by Marilyn and the family on their long trip. Over the next few days we drove home down the coast to complete a very pleasant adventure.

Perth, the Nullarbor and South Australia, 2005

To attend a College of Surgeons conference I had planned to take our Subaru Forester on the train to Perth and drive home. Unfortunately, the car was 25 mm too high to be taken on the train on the Sydney to Adelaide leg, so we decided to drive across the Hay Plains. Our first overnight stop was at Balranald. By chance I saw a flyer on the bedroom door advertising Mungo Lakes National Park so we decided to divert through there the following day. It is about a hundred kilometres off the main highway and the roads are rough and dusty. The "lake" is a former anabranch or diversion of the Murrumbidgee River, dry for millennia. These ancient lakes are characterised by flat bottoms and rimmed on the northern and eastern sides by ancient sand dunes, formed by then prevailing winds.

The park entrance is near the old sheep station buildings and contains some simple introductory posters. Nearby is the semi-derelict shearing shed, interesting in itself. There are also some self-service cabins available but no other amenities. The main points of interest are accessed by driving across the old lakebed for a couple of miles to reach the ancient dunes, the site of Aboriginal camps thought to be at least 30,000 years old. Successive erosion of the old dune structure reveals middens and old fire pits, sufficiently well preserved to give an excellent sense of some of the old campsites and their inhabitants enjoying feasts of the fish caught back in the days when the lakes held water. This was the site of discovery of the skeleton of Mungo woman, later followed by other skeletal remains of a people perhaps antedating the current Aboriginal race. It is a spiritual place, remote, simple and moving. Unfortunately, the flies were so numerous and aggressive that lunch was limited to a small tin of cold baked beans each, shovelled in quickly to thwart most of the dipterous competition.

That night we had a reservation in an historic Mildura hotel by the Murray River. The main attraction was Piero DiStefano's restaurant, situated in the original cellar of the Grand Hotel. The great man was not present but it was an excellent dinner with a degustation of numerous courses, some fine wines, and excellent service provided by attractive hospitality students from the local TAFE.

An uneasy sleep preceded an uneventful drive to Adelaide to join the train. The Indian Pacific has a couple of car-carrying wagons at the end and you have to get there early to load the car. That train trip is always memorable, leaving Adelaide late in the afternoon, taking most of the following day to cross the Nullarbor plain, stopping in Kalgoorlie late at night and reaching Perth the next morning. Our car was filthy from the locomotives' diesel exhausts which had played over it for a couple of thousand kilometres, so our first stop was to a carwash. I had opened the front seat windows to fold in the rear-view mirrors and then forgotten to close them before we went through the car wash. It only took one or two squirts of detergent foam and some animated shouting from Marilyn for me to rapidly close the windows.

After the conference we spent a couple of weeks to drive home, going in easy stages through the Margaret River area and stopping first at the south-west corner of the continent at Augusta. That was memorable for an unusually fierce storm making for a wild night. A little further north, at Busselton, there were destructive tornados. The coastal trip along the South-Western highway took us through impressive remnant forest, agricultural country, and further vineyards, eventually getting to Albany. From Esperance we made the short journey north to Norseman to prepare for our long trip across the Australian

Bight. The trip is well worthwhile. The roads are all paved now although their condition varies. Because we had plenty of time, we took every opportunity to leave the main road and see whatever tourist attractions were available on the high coastal cliffs of the Great Australian Bight. There is very little settlement except for the Road Houses, which are sited about every hundred kilometres and include fuel pumps, a very simple service area for food and groceries, and sometimes a little accommodation. Because water is scarce and mostly confined to rainfall, it is provided very sparingly to travellers. We stopped in Ceduna overnight. The ruins of the old Telegraph Station are largely buried by shifting sands. From there we deviated down to the tip of the Eyre Peninsula and Port Lincoln.

Some backtracking next day took us to the small seaside village of Coffin Bay for lunch. It was well outside holiday period but we found a small restaurant and an open-air table. Our only fellow diners were a couple of suited gentlemen, perhaps the local estate agents without much work to do but with an evident appreciation of the local produce. The oysters are justly famed and went down well with some Clare Valley Riesling. A drowsy afternoon drive through grassfire-devastated farmland led to rusty Whyalla for our night stop.

Becoming impatient to get home, we pushed on next day beyond Adelaide, into Western Victoria and through the Mallee. Working our way generally nor-east we came upon the striking outcrops of the Grampians and stopped overnight in that region and spent the next day sightseeing. With the motivation of homecoming we headed up the Newell Highway to end this marvellous trip encompassing the long-distance train, some very long road sections, many scenic areas which we had not seen before and the moving experience of Lake Mungo.

Other road trips

Our road trips usually lasted only several days to a week or so. That was enough to make many forays into both the North and South Coast, Victoria and Queensland. We preferred to take it easy, investigating side roads and any promising places of interest. Avoiding school holiday periods, we rarely booked ahead but found accommodation without much trouble. Once again, the free time of retirement allows plenty of flexibility and spontaneity.

Kimberley Coast with Oceanic Discoverer, 2014

21st of August, 2014 found us at Fort Hill Wharf in Darwin to enjoy our first glimpse of the Oceanic Discoverer, our cruise ship to explore the Kimberley coast. We had flown up that morning from Sydney. The following morning we reported at a quarter to eight for a friendly check-in and efficient embarkation.

Oceanic Discoverer

This little ship, 207 feet long, had been specially built in Cairns in 2005 for cruising the Northern Coast of Australia. There were 72 guests and 24 crew members. Our cabin was A05 on the bridge deck, immediately aft of the captain's own quarters. The accommodation was comfortable, including air-conditioning, a proper bathroom and toilet, with unlimited desalinated water for showers and laundry.

As well as the two big Caterpillar diesel main propulsion engines there was a separate auxiliary engine room with three smaller Caterpillar engines for generators, air conditioning, de-sal plant, waste management et cetera.

A key asset was the specially designed flat-bottomed barge Xplorer, big enough to seat all 72 guests plus several crew members, well shaded by a canopy, propelled by powerful twin outboard engines, and equipped with a retractable ramp at the bows to allow us to land easily on beaches. When not in use the craft was carried transversely across the stern of the ship, where it fitted perfectly on its special hydraulic powered cradle. This craft contributed enormously to the pleasure of the trip because it was so simple for us to embark and be transported quickly and comfortably ashore or afloat. It was supplemented by two or three Zodiac inflatable tenders which could take up to about eight or 10 passengers at a time.

The crew

Our skipper, Gary Wilson, was a tall, quiet chap who later warmed to reveal a friendly and informative manner. One moonless evening he gave a fascinating talk on the basics of celestial navigation. After the lecture we filed up to the sundeck and Gary had all the lights extinguished so he could demonstrate the more important stars and constellations which are often used for navigational sights.

Over breakfast one morning Gary had some good stories to tell. He had skippered the replica of Willem Janszoon's Duyfken (Little Dove) on many trips. It is an authentic reconstruction which he said, to my surprise, sailed so well to windward that there was seldom need to use the compulsorily installed diesel auxiliaries. At the time of our discussion this Duyfken project was in limbo because of lack of sponsorship and the ship remained in Holland. Gary had also skippered the New Endeavour replica several times.

The Expedition leader, Jamie Anderson, was often preoccupied with endless planning for shore excursions, safety, managing the efficient young crew, and herding the mostly older and far less biddable guests.

Much of the value and pleasure of our trip depended on the expert lecturers who accompanied each outing, gave some formal lectures and many impromptu discussions. Tim Harvey was a Marine Biologist and renowned sea-turtle expert and Damon Ramsey a general Naturalist. Both were talented and tireless photographers as well as friendly and helpful guides.

Our days' activities were planned around the tides and conditions, so that we saw and experienced whatever was most available. Some expeditions started early in the morning but more commonly we would have been at anchor by breakfast time, and then were free to join the shore expeditions using the Xplorer barge or Zodiacs, according to need. Usually we returned to the ship for a buffet lunch, perhaps moving on during the afternoon to some further point of interest. Most guests mustered at the bar for predinner drinks. That was the usual time for a formal debrief on the day's activities including a slideshow of our photographers' best efforts for the day and generally a more formal talk on some aspect of the History, Geology or wildlife of the Kimberley. While we slept, the ship was gently moved to its next anchorage.

Geology

The Kimberley region is geologically distinct from the rest of Australia and can be considered a residue left behind after separation of Australia from the Indian tectonic plate. It is mostly composed of sandstone or other sedimentary rocks with occasional volcanic basalt intrusions providing more fertile patches. Sandstone strata are absolutely horizontal in the north-east, becoming more deformed and fractured approaching Broome. Tides are very big, more than 10 metres, resulting in strong currents.

History

Pre-European history is mostly evidenced by the Aboriginal rock art, including both the Wandjina and Bradshaw styles of painting, numerous hand stencils, plus some examples of so-called “contact art” in which the Aborigines had depicted images of European style ships and humans apparently wearing hats, carrying firearms and using tobacco pipes. [Wandjinas are bold images of Creation spirits, often in red, yellow or black. Bradshaw or Gwion paintings are distinctively different, smaller, finer, and more realistic.] Early explorers of this coast include Matthew Flinders and Philip Parker King (see below). Inland, the early pioneers were pastoralists and later miners.

Flora and fauna

Biology is diverse, with abundant sea life but, oddly, few seabirds in the northerly part.

Birds included white bellied sea eagles, egrets, herons, and occasional brahman kites. We saw quite a few smaller reptiles, although on this trip we saw only a few crocodiles.

At low tide there were numerous cute bug-eyed little mud skippers hunting their smaller prey on the mudflats.

At sea there were numerous whales, sharks, turtles and other larger animals as well as an increasing number of seabirds as we approached Broome.

Notable landings and sites

Of the numerous shore excursions and landings which we made during the 10 days, some of the more notable included:

King George River, which we traversed all the way to the twin waterfalls at its head.

Mitchell Falls, which we visited by a Bell Jet Ranger helicopter, aviation's answer to the Land Cruiser. Taking off from the beach, we cruised at up to about 2000 feet over the mouth of the Hunter River to gain the plateau, a dry landscape of rocks, rocky shelves and outcrops and some thinly wooded savannah. Even in the dry season the Mitchell Falls looked very good, with many cascades falling through various levels. We landed at a bush camp for a few minutes to refuel. Our return flight took us straight back towards the west, passing over our ship swinging at anchor, to land back on the beach.

Naturalists' Island. Organisation for our sunset barbecue was superb. After drinks taken while sitting in folding chairs on the beach, we queued for a generous dinner with two kinds of sausages, fish, chicken, kangaroo steak, pork belly and the trimmings. Everybody's cameras clicked simultaneously as the sun set. As the tide came in we broke camp and quickly returned to the ship for desserts.

Our shore expedition next day was to Careening Cove, a spot where the explorer Phillip Parker King had beached his cutter "Mermaid" for repairs in 1818. King, born on Norfolk Island, was a Royal Navy officer who, among many other exploits, made four exploratory expeditions around the Australian coastline, to "fill in the gaps" left by Matthew Flinders. The Cove is a fertile little area of basalt soil, with cycads, bauhinia, and the ancient Boab tree in the bark of which the Mermaid crew had carved the ship's name. Somewhat incongruously, the powers-that-be have encircled the ancient tree, rather the worse for wear but still alive, with the ship's name legible, with an elevated walkway, complete with an array of informative old photographs and posters.

Prince Regent River. This was a long run up the mighty river, and we had to queue behind a couple of rival tour groups which had arrived before us. It was worth waiting for the beautiful experience of our turn at the Cascade. Our Xplorer barge nosed right up to the rock ledge and our extroverts jumped ashore for a forceful cool shower directly under the waterfall.

On Langgi Beach next morning we were greeted by the local mob of Aborigines. Their main spokesman was tall, eloquent and persuasive. They would have liked to sell some of their paintings. These were well executed but the prices, up to $1500, seemed a bit steep. I think they sold one or two. At low tide we were able to enter, one by one, an extraordinary cave, richly embellished with wall paintings including "contact art", probably depicting Dutch visitors.

At low tide this was a remarkable and beautiful area of broad sand beaches, red bluffs, deep green foliage, the gorge with little creeks entering it, and a remarkable group of eroded sandstone columns, said by the Aborigines to be their ancestors, including the chief and his wife on a battlefield. Assuming this yarn was true, the battle had left plenty of dead!

As we left, our hosts staged a smoking ceremony for our benefit. A little fire was set, then lit by the maître d' using his BIC cigarette lighter. Some green acacia leaves were added to provide the smoke, through which we dutifully filed to receive the good wishes of the elders and a daub of ochre on the forehead.

Montgomery Reef: At low tide next morning we visited Montgomery Reef, a broad area of coral reefs some 20km offshore and about 400km^2 in area. As the tide ebbs and the reef is exposed, a huge volume of water streams outward from the central lagoon in vast sheets, runnels and torrents, converging in a central gutter which they call The River. Our Xplorer and the Zodiacs ran for several kilometres up this river as it narrowed and finally shoaled. There were various seabirds feasting on the fish in the reef pools. Turtles were very numerous – a big black head appears, ducks, and reappears, then with a swirl the turtle dives and swims onwards. This complex of coral reefs is so unusual a spectacle, so visually attractive – a marvellous thing to have seen.

Horizontal Waterfalls: At slack water we could motor through the falls area and view Cyclone Creek, a traditional storm refuge for the area. The landforms were interesting; basically of sandstone but interspersed with softer conglomerates, siltstone, and mudstones. The narrow walls of the Horizontal Waterfalls had been excised by erosion of these softer rock formations.

Next day the ebb tide was right for us to enjoy the spectacle of the Horizontal Waterfalls. A memorable experience! Our Zodiacs took parties of about eight at a time. We needed to hang on as we enjoyed the bumpy ride against the outrushing tide. It all lasted only a few minutes before we turned around and coasted back on the torrent.

The Lecepides: This offshore sandy reef area was extraordinary for the myriad seabirds of all sorts accompanied by their chicks. Bosun birds were most abundant. There are also numerous turtles and both reef sharks and shovel-nosed sharks. The overwhelming impression was of the multitude of handsome, cheeky, uninhibited birds, after we had seen very few seabirds for the past nine days.

Yampi Sound: The eroded, complex, intricately folded and broken rock formations were the main point of interest. The now-abandoned iron ore mines on Koolan and Iron Islands and their disused loading jetties were interesting in themselves but also because they were the first man-made artefacts other than cruise ships that we had seen in eight days.

On our final evening we enjoyed the traditional Captain's cocktail party.

Just before dawn the ship lay stationary off Cable Beach, then entered Broome harbour just after sunrise. After breakfast we disembarked and said our farewells to the crew before taking our coach to Cable Beach resort.

A day's sojourn in Broome, an easy flight to Perth and a relaxing return to Sydney on the Indian Pacific Train: a perfect coda to an outstanding and informative cruise on the Oceanic Discoverer.

Comment: This trip on a purpose-built coastal expedition trip exemplified some of the best aspects of travel:

The ship and its tenders performed perfectly.

An outstanding crew contributed so much. The Captain and deck officers and engineer were friendly but always professional and effective. A clever strategy had the deck crew and hotel staff change tasks halfway through the cruise, keeping the youngsters happy and on the ball.

The "tour" staff were excellent. Director Jamie Anderson planned excursions to suit tides and conditions, ran a tight ship, was unofficial casualty officer for minor injuries and illnesses, and was a fine overall Tour Leader. Guides Tim Harvey and Biologist Damon Ramsey were just what we needed, hosting the shore parties, photographing wildlife and points of interest, debriefing each day's expeditions, and giving really informative lectures on Geology, History, Geography, Biology and many other titbits to inform and delight us.

Whale Watching, 2016 and 2017

(What is the whale watching while she is watching the whale watchers watching?)

In the winter of 2016 we decided to escape to the north and enjoy watching the whales in Hervey Bay. Marilyn had been there a few years earlier with her sister Roslyn and was keen to repeat the experience. We allowed three days to drive there and three days at the Mantra Hotel, right on the waterfront. Choosing the best-looking weather forecast, we signed up for a day-long boat trip. This was a good choice because the round trip to the best areas takes a good two or three hours, leaving not much time for whale watching if you take only a half-day trip. We got lucky. It was a perfect day, clear weather, smooth water, and after a while the whales turned up and put on an amazing show. We had often seen them from the shore but being right beside them on a small boat is another experience altogether. They seemed to enjoy watching us and playing like kittens. It was such a marvellous performance that our skipper stayed for hours beyond his normal departure time. There was even a new-born calf nearby although we didn't get close enough to see much of it.

The 2016 whale watching trip was such a success that we repeated it in 2017. Once again it was a delight, but I do not think we will repeat it in 2018.

Overseas trips with Owen

There were some extraordinary overseas trips with Owen Johnstone-Donnet and St. James Rail: Japan; Scandinavia; and Isle of Man, Wales, Cornwall and the Hebrides.

Japan, 2005

The "Autumn Leaves" trip to Japan in October 2005 did not begin auspiciously. Guide Bob Dickie met us at the check-in with the news that our incoming plane had been held up, so our flight was deferred till next morning. A typically indifferent Qantas sent us off to the Mercure hotel without making proper bookings. Eventually someone found a buffet dinner and a room. Next morning was no more promising as the buses were late and the check-in queues monstrous, so we eventually left 45 minutes late. Things looked up as our replacement 747 was only about 10% full, providing plenty of room to exercise, plenty of free Asahi beer and plenty of seats for a nap.

Order was restored when we were met by Owen at Narita airport. The fast train to Tokyo and a connecting commuter train transferred us to our hotel at Kawasaki. Next morning, after a traditional Japanese breakfast of miso, fish, etc, we headed downtown for an extensive walk to find our land legs and get attuned to the go-go rhythm of Japan. In a park we bumped into a TV film crew shooting a children's gardening show, then found some fellows drumming in the park. A couple of derelicts lay asleep by the pathway, one with his socks drying on a nearby bush. A long hot walk took us to the imposing Emperor's Palace, complete with drawbridge, on to spectacular fountains and back to the station to meet the remainder of our tour group who had flown in that morning. We had lunch in a dining area called Kitchen Street located in a subway beneath the railway station. Not much room wasted there. There we met Cam and Janet Alexander and shared a salad and a drink.

We later became good friends with the Alexanders who had a house at Killcare Heights. Back at the Kawasaki hotel we had barely time to clean up and join the group for an excellent dinner of salmon, rice, and a French white wine. We were really tired!

So it continued for nearly four hectic weeks of trains old and new, shinkansen bullet trains, tilt trains that banked around unbanked bends, sleeper trains, ordinary trains, commuter trains, rail motors, monorails, trams, cable cars, taxis, minibuses, in a blur of activity and sensational discoveries, all coordinated superbly by Owen, his mother Pam, and guide Bob Dickie. We crisscrossed the length of the Japanese islands back-and-forth, over bridges, under tunnels and on an occasional ferry. Endless shrines, temples, pagodas and castles.

Japan really is overwhelming; it is almost impossible to nominate individual highlights. A breath-taking "Wow!" moment on rounding a tall hedge to reveal the Golden Pagoda in Kyoto? The orderliness and efficiency of all services? The official politeness, cleanliness and tidiness of public services? The personal politeness and friendliness and helpfulness of everyday people? The inefficiency of having so many meet-and-greet people in the big stores? Pure make-work! Another delight was on our final night in Akashi, when after walking around the city for some hours we chose a small "Red Lantern" tempura bar for dinner. (The red lantern refers to the distinguishing lamp out the front, not the activities within.) We had almost finished our dinner of tempura, omelette and beer when a pair of nearby fellow diners sent an extra dish to us as a gift. They were optical engineers, visiting the town for their work, out on the town and already generously lubricated. Our conversation was limited by the obvious language difficulties but they were friendly and inquisitive. The proprietor joined in and informed us that his daughter was studying in Australia on the Gold Coast. After a new bottle of sake fuelled several toasts to our International friendship, we escaped.

Because the weather remained warm we never did see many autumn leaves but it was an extraordinary trip.

Scandinavia, 2007

Second of August 2007 found us roaring and rattling above the Siberian tundra in a venerable Finnair MD-11 aircraft, maybe a recycled freighter. Helsinki first stop, in time for a lengthy lakeside walk in the long afternoon. So began our St James rail tour of Scandinavia.

We had not visited the Baltic region before this, and it is a marvellous destination, varied, scenically spectacular, mostly sophisticated, comfortable, and civilised.

Finland was perhaps the most distinctive of these Nordic countries. Outside the main cities it is still thinly populated, with agriculture and forestry predominating. Dominated by Russia throughout most of the 19th and early 20th centuries, it still has a Russian feel to it, with lakeside dachas and their saunas, timber or stone churches which look Orthodox but are often Lutheran, and a somewhat taciturn people.

After we had enjoyed the modern city of Helsinki and its more traditional surrounds, our trip took us partly by waterways but mostly by train northward to the Arctic Circle. Santa Claus village was a disappointing tourist trap, but I did not really expect to meet the bearded old fraud there in person. One memorable highlight was an outdoors zoo. A very personable young guide showed us around. At the beginning it was a let-down because the nocturnal animals could not be seen and the birds were confined to a smallish aviary, but the big animals, especially the polar bears, brown bears and reindeer were excellent and the lynx really spectacular.

An overnight sleeper train took us back to Helsinki, from where we took a large car ferry for the two-hour trip to Tallinn, the well preserved ancient capital of Estonia. Our guide was a fitness freak who insisted on walking or jogging us briskly about two kilometres uphill on a hot afternoon to the old city. This really was a charming mediaeval place with separate top and bottom towns, old Guild houses and churches. A "Greek" wedding was in progress at the beautiful Orthodox church on the hill, with the chanting priest, guests in various folk dress and modern suits, all standing for the ceremony. A ridiculous white stretch limo stood at the doors.

We walked more slowly back to the waterfront where Ron White and I found life-saving beer while Marilyn and Toni enjoyed infused tea and cakes.

We boarded our overnight ferry to Stockholm. A flat sea and gentle propeller harmonics, after a busy day, all contributed to sound sleep.

Stockholm is a beautiful city with several good museums among its attractions. The Royal Vasa Museum was a truly superb display of the old warship, reclaimed from the mud after hundreds of years. The following morning was taken up by the Nordic Museum, and in the afternoon we enjoyed a ferry excursion through the nearby archipelago, admiring traditional and modern waterside houses and the few recreational craft.

Our trip north through Sweden over several days mostly utilised modern trains but some sectors were devoted almost entirely to tourism, with frequent informal stops for points of interest such as a photo opportunity, the top of a mountain pass, or even a bear's lair in the forest. The countryside was very attractive with forests of birch and fir, or dairy farms with prosperous farmhouses and some cultivation.

The following day took us across the high country and the iron mining precinct of Kiruna, after which we crossed the border into Norway, eventually arriving at the iron port of Narvik.

Next day's great coach trip down the west coast of Norway from Narvik to Bodo – six hours' worth of driving spread over 12 hours - was visually exhausting. Some of the highlights:

- A lowering sky with occasional drizzle
- Rugged ice-carved mountains almost treeless towards their top
- Moss covered rocks and sparse trees at road level
- Lunch. The fish stew turned out to be cold salmon with sweet potato and turnip mash, plus salad with a couple of white wines
- Our first sight of a troll, waving his flag while standing in a waterfall, enjoying a lovely view down the fjord. (Trolls are a semi-serious part of Nordic folklore, often represented by doll-like piles of flat stones either naturally occurring or man-made and presenting a quaintly humanoid silhouette)
- Mountains are formed of schist or gneiss with prominent bands of quartz.
- As we rolled into Fauske we began to see outcrops of marble and limestone, and in the town we stopped at the quarry where they mine the local Fauske Rose marble. Our fellow guest, Barney Elliston, gave a fine talk on the geology.

- Lars, our nicotine addicted driver, recommended we visit the famed Saltstrom maelstrom. At first it was a disappointing anti-climax but the tide finally revved up so the water was ebbing at least 10 knots, forming most impressive whirlpools. As I walked back to the bus a small freighter shot through the narrows with the tide and was out of sight in a few minutes.

By train from Trondheim south to Andalnse, then on to Oslo involved a spectacular series of alternating fjords and uplands. The scenery and geology were captivating. There was plenty to see in Oslo including:

- The Fram Museum, dedicated to the polar adventures of Nansen, Amundsen and others
- A movie on the coast of Norway featuring spectacular helicopter shots
- The Kon Tiki Museum
- The Viking Ships Museum featuring many well preserved remnants of the great longships
- A huge sculpture garden showing the works of Gustav Vigelund. I got a photograph of the bust of Charles Darwin, which was nice because I happened to be reading "On the Origin of Species".

A couple more days of train travel took us to Bergen and its surrounds. Bergen is a very ancient port city and contains great museums, forts and warehouses of the Hanseatic League, the Mediaeval trading empire of towns and Guilds, embracing the Rhineland, the Baltic area, the Lowlands and much of southern England, long before the consolidation of modern Germany. Bergen was also our port of departure on the Hurtigruten ferry to the north.

These ferries conduct a "mail run" up the west coast of Norway and round the North Cape to Kirkenes, adjacent to the Russian border. Our ship, the MS Finnmarken was one of the newer ones, built in 2002, with 620 beds and a passenger capacity of 1000 in all. It was about 140 M in length and 15,500 tons – a tidy size, beautifully built and maintained. As well as carrying passengers – both locals and tourists – it made detours into most of the fjords to act as the supply ship for their small cities. It is a most impressive and efficient service. At each port the ship ties alongside, opens a huge door on its side, and unloads and on-loads cargo with forklifts, while the passengers are free to take tourist trips ashore.

The total journey took six nights, and every day was full of glorious Fjordland scenery.

Beyond North Cape our voyage ended at Kirkenes. We enjoyed a day of local sightseeing, out to the Russian and Finnish borders, then took a late evening flight south to Oslo.

Next day was an excellent train trip to Gothenburg in Sweden. Here most of our tour group broke away and only a few of us continued for the rail trip from Malmo in Sweden across the great Oresund Bridge and a tunnel to Copenhagen in Denmark. We had particularly arranged this extension of the tour to visit our friends Lissi and Stein with whom we had shared good times in Abu Dhabi.

At Lissi's suggestion we spent the first day enjoying the sights of the city and the harbour as tourists, and the next day took the train up the east coast to lunch with her near Helsingore (Elsinore). The Castle dates from 1500 or so and is still used for occasional receptions and for stagings of Hamlet - it was, after all, his old house. Huge. We visited the casements which were dark and dank, the chapel which was elegantly beautiful, and the Royal Chambers - two floors of extraordinary rooms. Only a few furnishings remain but very many tapestries, some paintings and ornate ceilings. A hearty "traditional Danish" seafront lunch ensued and we visited Lissi's own house, an apartment in a rebuilt barn. She took us back to our train.

Next morning, apart from the pain of paying for our laundry, wine, minibar and phone bills (ouch!), it was time to trundle our bags one last timc through the sex shops to catch our train for the airport and the trip home.

Finnair to Hong Kong, quick shower and a fresh shirt, change to Cathay Pacific, and an uneventful flight to Sydney.

A great trip!

South-Western UK and Hebrides Tour in 2012

Isle of Man

Our 2012 St James Rail tour to the western parts of the British Isles began with a Virgin Rail trip from Euston Station to Liverpool. That was our first encounter with the Pendolino ("Pendulum"), an Italian-designed, Spanish-built tilt train offering a very fast and smooth ride in comfortable and agreeable seating.

We took the ferry to Douglas on the Isle of Man and trundled our bags along the elegant promenade to our hotel. Our first full day on the island was taken up by a ride in an old steam train to Port Erin near the southern tip of the island. The most important site visited was the House of Keys, the original Parliament of the Isle of Man. An interactive hologram displayed a pretend debate of the Council while we sat around their original boardroom table. The island, although now part of the United Kingdom, retains its self-government to this day.

Next day was memorable for the use of so many transport modes:

- Walk to the far south end of the promenade
- Horse tram back along three kilometres of the promenade
- An electric tram to Laxey where we climbed its immense water wheel
- Electric tram to the 620m summit of Snaefell and back
- Tram onward to Ramsey
- Double-decker bus to Peel
- Then a marvellous circuit of the Isle of Man Tourist Trophy motorbike race track aboard a motor tricycle.

We had seen the flyer for IOM Trikes in our hotel lobby, and Owen organised for us to be picked up by them at Peel. We were not dressed for the occasion but our host kitted us out in strong waxed cotton black coats, and helmets fitted with intercom. We were seated side-by-side behind our driver, whose seat was that of a conventional motorcycle with long chopper style front forks. With a 1200cc car engine, there was more than enough power, but we toddled along sedately without exceeding 80kph [The Tourist Trophy has been run annually since 1907, with some nine years missed due to the two World Wars. Modern riders complete the 61km course at average speeds well above 200kph, reaching 300kph on the straight, hard to believe when the race is run on ordinary narrow roads through village streets.] There were plenty of stops along the way for us to see points of interest and to be told stories of the big bike race. A Boys' Own Adventure for me!

Wales

Next day was a longer ferry trip back to the mainland at Morecambe Bay in Wales. Much of our time in Wales was cool and drizzly, but that did not prevent our enjoyment of numerous scenic trips on old-narrow gauge tramways, often of only about 60cm gauge, and generally drawn by small historic steam locomotives.

Until recently this area of Wales was the world centre of slate mining. We saw plenty of the old pits, as well as the work sheds in which thc rocks were cleaved into individual slates for transport all over the world. The industry has more recently been undercut by the Chinese substitute. On one of the slate tours I noted as we climbed into the forest in increasing drizzle that it was a slate grey day with slate grey rain amid slate grey clouds beside waste slate roads with houses whose roofs, walls, and floors were all built of slate.

Next day a steep rail climb took us almost to the summit of Mount Snowdon. The journey certainly was picturesque, until we were engulfed by the dense fog covering the uppermost third of the mountain. Denied the famous outlook from the top, we contented ourselves with a cup of coffee instead.

Pembrokeshire had long been the most "English" part of Wales. At St David's we joined the quarter past eleven service, a high Anglican "bells and smells" affair, enlivened by a very fine choir with an outstanding soprano soloist. An unusual tourist spot was an old corn mill powered by the high tides of the area. The mill wheel, set in a dam across a small estuary, powered the multi-storied mill: the "gear" floor which held the main mechanism, the "stone" floor which housed the grinding stones and winnowing apparatus, a bin floor for the unground wheat and several smaller machines powered by belt transmissions. It would have been a powerful, reliable and effective industrial application of its day.

Devon and Cornwall

To get to the South Coast of England we went a long way around, Cardiff to London Paddington Station, then changing to a fast train to Exeter in Devon. A couple of other trains and a rail motor led us to Barnstaple.

Next day was a bus trip west along the Bristol Channel, stopping at Tintagel, Boscastle and Port Isaac, known to long-suffering Doc Martin watchers as Portwenn. Padstow presented a cold and steady drizzle. In need of a place to eat lunch, we were allowed to use the lawn of a hotel as long as we bought a drink. Here we enjoyed Rick Stein's takeaway fish and chips, somewhat cool and congealed, washed down with beer or wine to taste, as we stood around in our damp clothes and squishy shoes.

In Cornwall our lodging was at Carbis Bay Hotel, just west of St Ives. Expeditions included a chilly and foggy jaunt to Land's End, the most enjoyable part of which was a subterranean cable station dating from World War II. This was the site where the original transatlantic cable had come ashore.

Another worthwhile experience was the Eden Project, a very impressive engineering feat creating in effect several gigantic terraria of inflatable greenhouses within a huge old quarry. It was well worth the visit although some of the Greenie propaganda was intrusive.

Scotland and the Hebrides

A comfortable Virgin Rail trip back to London and an overnight sleeper took us to Inverness. Next day's rail motor journey westward across Scotland was a scenic feast of lochs, forests, and mountains before arriving at Lochailsh. Thence we crossed the bridge to the Isle of Skye and settled in our converted hunting lodge hotel for the next couple of nights.

Isle of Skye is romantic territory for those of us with Scottish blood, who had grown up with the legends of Bonnie Prince Charlie. It is a ruggedly beautiful place with black-faced sheep and some long-horned Highland cattle, the dramatic Cuillin mountains, and rugged multicoloured "tartan" cliffs.

A couple of days later we took the ferry across the Minch to the Isle of Harris. I enjoyed watching a display of hand-loom weaving, which they still use to manufacture the beautiful Harris Tweed suitings. An afternoon bus trip took us north through the bleak countryside to the evocative town of Stornoway. This is an ancient and strategic port with substantial quayside buildings.

Next day we visited Callaway, interesting for its stone circles and old Fort building, and for the village of refurbished black houses in various states of repair. These are the low walled solid stone houses with a thatch retained by cables weighted down by huge stones to retain the roof during the winter gales. We looked through one of the black houses. One end was reserved for the cow byre, while a primitive little kitchen had a small smoky peat fire smouldering on a simple central hearth on the floor beneath an opening in the roof for the smoke. Curtained sleeping quarters were at the opposite end from the cows.

Peat was everywhere on the hillsides and in the houses, still used for cooking and rudimentary heating. Stone is the ubiquitous building material for walls of the farmhouses, outbuildings, fences and animal pens. Each dwelling had one long thin field only about a chain [say 10m] wide, which must only have supported the most meagre living as there was not much room for cultivation or grazing – it was simply too small, especially in that hard clime. These are the farms now largely held by "crofters" – often absent landlords.

We drove through the southernmost part of the Isles of Lewis and North and South Harris which are far more mountainous, smaller but similar to the

Cuillens of Skye. The sheep have it to themselves. By the time we got to the south side of the island of South Harris the scene was of white sandy beaches and dunes, saltmarsh, and more numerous houses. At Rodel we visited the mediaeval church of St Clements. A very old collie dog who was guarding the entrance reluctantly admitted us, then enjoyed a halting sacrilegious piddle on an interior wall. In the churchyard we found a McAulay gravestone dated 1730, also a McLennan and plenty of McLeods. And it was a Roman Catholic Church! [The reason for this snide comment is that my maternal grandmother was a McAulay and claimed to have descended from the Isle of Skye but nobody on Skye could recall that surname. Rodel was the first place where we came across it during this trip. And Gran was a bigoted anti-Catholic.]

At a bird reserve in marshlands at Benbecula not many birds were to be seen but Marilyn acted the galah in her pink wind cheater.

Over on South Uist it was flatter with innumerable fresh lakes - this is famous angling territory. It looks incredibly fertile - mainly grazing on broad fields.

Fifth of July was one of the best days of this trip. The lazy start at 9.45 AM was a good omen. We gathered at the waterfront for a short boat trip out to the "Castle on a Rock" – the traditional fortress of the Clan MacNeill. The fortress occupied the whole rock. Having been refurbished between the Wars by a wealthy American McNeil, the castle was well presented but a really damp, dank place. I particularly liked the motto on the McNeil crest: "Buiadh no bas (Victory or Death)".

Back on shore, we took the Herring Walk along the open quay where a bustling fishery used to thrive on processing and pickling the herring for export until it was killed off by the world wars, fish poachers, overfishing, and the usual political fish troubles over sovereignty, quotas and tariffs.

A minibus took us to the north side of the island to visit Barra airport, which is in fact the broad shingle beach at low tide. As we had our lunch a small twin turbo Islander plane, probably about a 10-seater, landed on the beach, reloaded and took off.

Two ferry rides, transhipping at Oban, took us to the Isle of Mull. Its high peak, Ben More, of near 1000M, is bare near the top but lower down has more trees than we had seen for some time, with plenty of pine plantations. There is good grazing land with plenty of cattle and sheep.

The town of Tobermory occupies a very steep sidling, its bright coloured buildings clustered around a small bay. The hotel itself was also steep with four levels including our “Turret”, 82 steps in all, affording spectacular views over the Sound of Mull and the mainland hills beyond. First stop next day was Lachlan Macquarie’s mausoleum, a plain stone structure within a stone circle in the woods. It was moving to think of our eminent New South Wales Governor who had been buried here on his retirement estate, not far from his birth place on the tiny Isle of Ulva.

On to Torasay Castle, where we lunched alfresco. One surprise inside the castle was to find several watercolours which had been painted by Apsley Cherry-Garrard, the young member of Scott’s Antarctic expedition who wrote “The Worst Journey in the World” (One of the best books on Antarctic exploration, though).

Next day a boating trip around the north of the Island of Mull, in dark weather with some rain, strong north winds and moderate sea brought us to the tiny rocky island of Lunga, part of a small archipelago famed for its bird population. Docking was a crazy procedure involving a very unstable pontoon-cum-gangplank contraption, followed by a clamber over a shingle composed of loose half-metre diameter boulders, then a climb up a slippery steep muddy path to a halfway plateau with a few derelict ruins. A big colony of puffins occupied innumerable clifftop burrows. They are really cute, waddling little blokes with bright red feet and beaks and a white breast, and a very funny way of running and launching themselves off the cliff edge.

Onward to Staffa, where spectacular basalt formations form flutes in various orientations, a Giant’s Causeway, and a narrow walk around the base of the cliff to Fingal’s Cave. This was an enthralling grotto with its deep clear water, blue jellyfish, a high fluted vault, and amazing echoes. Very cold!

Then to Iona with its impressively big Mediaeval Monastery which had been well restored in the 20th century, and the nunnery which remains derelict. Marilyn bought a few skeins of multicoloured wool for Alison and herself. We then had a strategic stop at the pub for a Tobermory 10 year old malt whiskey with a splash of water — warming!

It was then a short boat ride back to the Island of Mull to join our coach for a two-hour drive home.

A hearty Scottish breakfast prepared us for the ferry and our farewell to the Hebrides. Less than an hour later we were back in Oban, lunching on a sandwich and a prawn and crayfish salad, accompanied by an ale and a Hardy’s Chardonnay. Just time to take the train for Glasgow.

We had second-class seats but it was a scenic trip along lochs, and through valleys with plenty of fertile pastures and an occasional red deer or two. Some of the towns we passed included Taynuilt, Lochaber, Dalmalley, Crianlarich, Garelochead and Helensburgh. By a quarter past three we were entering the Glasgow suburbs with the usual regrets on leaving the outback. It was starting to rain.

Back in London we had some funny adventures changing trains at Euston, buying new tickets from machines, queueing on the wrong side of escalators; all the errors of new chums in a strange land. Victoria Station was less of a shambles. From there we caught the seven o'clock in the evening express to Gatwick with a shuttle to the North Terminal and an easy walk to our Sofitel Airport Hotel.

Next morning started with a good English breakfast (but the Scottish ones were even better). Pack up, check out, easy stroll to check in for our flight. By now we were both pretty drowsy - long days, and the usual post-trip let down.

That's when things went bad! Very heavy rain storms and bad weather delayed our take-off by two hours so we missed our connections in Dubai and were stranded there at two in the morning. A not particularly engaged or competent passenger (non-) services chap, probably a Somali, took a good hour but finally rebooked us on a quarter past ten flight that morning and secured a room at an airport hotel with limo transfer. After a short sleep and a welcome shower we were back in our same clothing to return to the airport to board our new Airbus A380 and left on time.

Summary

Owen Johnstone-Donnet and St James Rail really excelled themselves on this long and complex trip to the western parts of England and Wales and the Hebrides. We crammed in an amazing variety of experiences, trips, food, history, and mostly good fellowship. Days were full and long but we kept up and enjoyed every minute of it.

Afterword

Dear reader, if you ever wonder why authors so commonly nominate their spouse for the first position in the acknowledgements, ask the spouse.

Writing is largely a solitary occupation, often tedious and sometimes frustrating. My wife of sixty-six years, Marilyn has encouraged me through ages of these fragmentary literary efforts. In our case, she also supported me through sharing the exacting and taxing travails of a pioneering surgeon. Without her help the life could not have been lived and the story would never have been written.

Next honour goes to professional writers, Helen Menzies and Alison Handmer. Both are journalists and teachers, and both are supportive of their less talented acquaintances.

My participation in one of Helen's early life writing courses started the process. She has a particular skill and great patience in cajoling her mostly senior pupils into transforming experience into written words. She read this manuscript in its earlier versions many times and specifically suggested a way to resolve the biographer's conundrum of how to combine a chronological story with many topics which either do not fit in the timeline or else deserve their separate essay.

My son, John, and I often share ideas, but my daughter, Alison, has contributed decisively to the nuts and bolts of turning the manuscript into a publishable book, and presiding over its production. And she is very persuasive.

Next I acknowledge the assistance of hundreds of colleagues, teachers, mentors and friends. Many are named in this story but many more contributed. This multitude includes not only family and fellow doctors, but nurses, technical and clerical people, employees, volunteers and others, even administrators and politicians. While I gladly accepted the Australian honour of the Order of Australia in 1995 in recognition of my service to paediatric cardiology and cardiac surgery, I readily acknowledge that this award was not mine alone. No complex endeavour achieved anything without a supportive professional and social environment.

Thanks to Royal Prince Alfred Museum and Archives.

As usual, my apologies for any inadvertent errors.

Beyond my power to state in words, I express my gratitude to all the patients who entrusted their care to me and my team; even more to the parents and families of the children on whom I operated.

Index of names and institutions

About the author

Children's heart surgeon Tim Cartmill AO was born in Grafton on the NSW north coast in 1933, and raised in the nearby rural community of Nymboida. A bookish child, encouraged by his family and the teacher of his one-room school, he became a boarder at the selective Hurlstone Agricultural High School in Sydney.

Tim entered the University of Sydney Medical School at the age of sixteen. After graduation he served as Resident Medical Officer and Registrar at Royal Prince Alfred Hospital where he developed a lasting interest in chest surgery, especially the newly evolving field of open heart operations.

Having qualified as a Fellow of the Royal Australasian College of Surgery, he was privileged to study heart surgery for three years in USA at Houston, Texas and Mayo Clinic in Minnesota, two of the world-leading centres of the time.

Tim returned to Australia with his young family. He joined the staff at Royal Prince Alfred Hospital and Royal Alexandra Hospital for Children in Sydney from the mid-1960s until 1997, later participating in the establishment of Westmead Children's Hospital.

His service to paediatric cardiology and cardiac surgery were recognised in 1995 when he received the Order of Australia.

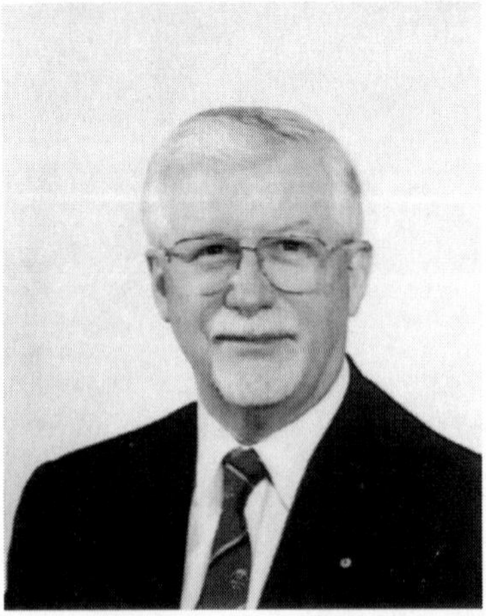

Having retired from active practice in Australia, Tim practised in Abu Dhabi in the United Arab Emirates from 1998 to 2001.

Professor Cartmill has helped train generations of Australian and International Heart surgeons and contributed to many overseas philanthropic surgical visits.

Other contributions included administrative, educational and political positions.

Understanding Life Backwards is an autobiography which also reflects on selected technical aspect of surgery, teaching, learning and mentorship, and the roles of colleagues, family and friends in a busy professional life. Finally, this book recounts many satisfactions of life in retirement, and muses on philosophy, retirement and aging.

About the publisher

Lorikeet Press publishes feel-good books for readers of all ages.

www.lorikeetpress.com

Made in United States
North Haven, CT
05 November 2026

21861532R00143